# *Heal*
# Your Body

## STEP BY STEP GUIDE TO THE

# ANTI-INFLAMMATORY DIET

## + 100 RECIPES TO NOURISH & REPAIR

**By Andre Parker**

# Other Books by Andre Parker

Please check out my other books also available on Amazon by visiting my Author's Page:

**amazon.com/author/andreparker.co**

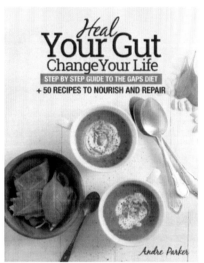

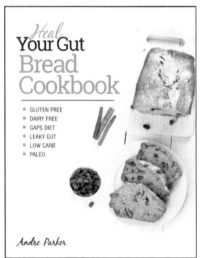

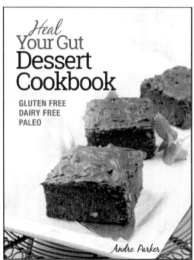

Facebook:     https://www.facebook.com/healyourguts/
Instagram:    https://www.instagram.com/andreparker.co/

If you enjoyed this book,
I'd appreciate it if you would leave a review.
Your feedback means the world to me so please do leave a review!

Simply visit: https://www.amazon.com/dp/B06Y63RD5K

# TABLE OF CONTENTS

# Introduction
## What is an Anti-Inflammatory Diet?

Anti-inflammatory diets have been in the spotlight for quite some time now as being a great diet to improve our overall health. There is a great deal of evidence that these diets reduce inflammation in the body and our chances of getting sick, whether with the common cold or a more serious illness, are therefore much lower. Whilst following an anti-inflammatory diet can help improve anyone's health, they are especially helpful for those of us who suffer from inflammatory conditions such as arthritis, gout, lupus and scleroderma to help to reduce the systemic inflammation that occurs with these conditions.

If you have ever heard of the saying, 'you are what you eat', this is entirely true. If you put processed, inflammation-causing foods into your body, you are going to cause inflammation, which is then going to result in unwanted reactions, such as digestive distress, skin conditions, mood disruptions and even disease. If you fuel your body with powerful inflammation fighting foods that are rich in phytonutrients and have the ability to fight disease, you are feeding your body what it needs to function at its most optimal level. An anti-inflammatory diet focuses on just that, feeding your body with the foods that it needs in order to thrive.

The anti-inflammatory diet is a diet full of wholesome, healthy and unprocessed foods. These wholesome foods act to naturally reduce the inflammation in your body and therefore prevent disease. There have been numerous research studies carried out on the benefits of anti-inflammatory diets. One study has shown that unresolved inflammation in the body has been linked to the early development of disease and argues that controlling inflammation should be 'a key future preventive and therapeutic target' ([1]). Another study indicated that consuming certain foods, such as: citrus fruits; tomatoes; dark, leafy greens; and wild-caught salmon, can fight disease-causing inflammation in the body ([2]).

So, you may be wondering what you would be eating on an anti-inflammatory diet. An anti-inflammatory diet is rich in healthy fats, particularly omega-3 fatty acids, which are not only great for combating inflammation, they are great for brain health as well. Foods high in omega-3 fatty acids include wild salmon, sardines, avocados, flaxseeds, hempseeds and walnuts. Fruits and vegetables should be enjoyed in abundance on an anti-inflammatory diet and provide the body with powerful antioxidants to fight off free radicals that are causing damage and inflammation to our organs. Herbs and spices are also commonly seen on an anti-inflammatory diet. Herbs and spices such as turmeric, garlic, ginger and green tea have been known to help to fight inflammation, and promote health, for centuries. These herbs and spices are also rich in bioflavonoids, which can help to reduce the amount of free radicals in the body. As far as proteins go, proteins such as grass-fed animal products are the protein of choice as opposed to grain-fed animal products that will produce more inflammation. Organic, pasture-raised eggs can also be enjoyed on an anti-inflammatory diet.

There are still so many delicious foods that can be consumed and incorporated into your everyday diet when following an anti-inflammatory way of eating. By eliminating foods that are processed, high in sugar, refined, grain-fed animal products, alcohol or contain excessive caffeine, you will be hugely helping to reduce the overall inflammation in your body.

# What is Inflammation?

When you think about inflammation, what comes to mind? For most, it's likely redness, swelling, heat, and pain but inflammation can stem from the inside of the body and is the culprit of nearly all disease seen today. Before we jump into talking about how you can make changes to your diet to help combat systemic inflammation, it's important to understand what is going on inside your body when inflammation is present. If you can understand what inflammation is and what's causing the inflammation you are well on your way to helping safeguard your body from inflammatory diseases.

The first thing to understand is that not all inflammation is bad. In fact, inflammation is part of the healing process and can help protect the body from both infection and disease. Acute inflammation such as when you get a wound helps that wound heal. The first stage of inflammation is called irritation which will then become inflammation followed by discharge of pus from a wound. Next, is the granulation stage which is where round masses of tissue form during the healing process (3). All you need to take away from this process is that without inflammation, wounds would never get the chance to heal. Acute inflammation can also be remembered by coming on suddenly, and signs and symptoms may appear to be pretty severe, but they generally only last a few days or in some cases a few weeks. Think bronchitis, a cut on the skin, or a sore throat. While acute inflammation can help, the body heal; inflammation becomes a problem when it becomes chronic.

Chronic inflammation lasts much longer than a few days. In fact, it can last months and even years. Chronic inflammation can occur as a result of an autoimmune reaction, a chronic irritant, or keeping that irritant that caused the inflammation in the first place in either your diet or your environment. Some of the conditions associated with chronic inflammation include asthma, rheumatoid arthritis, Crohn's disease, ulcerative colitis, and chronic peptic ulcers. Chronic inflammation can also lead to a handful of other diseases including certain cancers which is why it's so important to address the inflammation at its source.

The bottom line is that inflammation over the long term can be devastating to one's health. Making dietary and lifestyle chances are an imperative part of getting inflammation under control and with inflammation being the root cause of nearly all disease we all have to do our part to protect our health with the food choices we make.

Now that you know a little bit more about inflammation and the difference between acute inflammation and chronic inflammation, let's take a look at their causes.

# CAUSES OF CHRONIC INFLAMMATION

*Diet*

There are many dietary choices than can lead to inflammation. Refined carbohydrates, pesticides that you find in conventionally grown produce, sugar, factory farmed animal and dairy products that are pumped with hormones, antibiotics, and steroids, processed and fried foods, rancid oils such as vegetable oils, food additives, artificial sweeteners, excessive alcohol intake, gluten.

*Lifestyle Factors*

While diet plays a large role in the inflammatory process, your lifestyle choices do as well. A sedentary lifestyle has been shown to continue to conditions that are caused by inflammation such as obesity, and even diabetes. Physical inactivity, could also very well be a leading cause of disease and disability (4). If you work a desk job or are not as active as you would like to be, incorporating exercise into your lifestyle is super important for overall health.

*Sleep Habits*

Research has pointed to a lack of quality sleep as a cause of increased inflammation. Sleep habits are incredibly important not just for your physical health but your mental health as well. If you struggle with getting enough sleep at night, making dietary changes may help you more than you may think and exercising early in the day can also play a role.

# THE SOLUTION TO CHRONIC INFLAMMATION

Now that you know some of the key triggers of inflammation, let's review what you can do with your diet to turn inflammation around. When talking about food, it's all about removing those inflammatory foods and bulking up on anti-inflammatory food choices.

*What Are Anti-Inflammatory Foods?*

Adopting an anti-inflammatory diet means incorporating foods that are known to help the body fight inflammation. It also means eliminating the foods that trigger inflammation and reducing the toxic load on our body. If you really think about all the foods our bodies are exposed to on a daily basis it's no wonder inflammation runs rampant. Pesticide, herbicides, hormones, antibiotics, steroids, and food additives are hidden in the foods we eat and if we don't pay attention to exactly what we are eating we can fall victim to the inflammatory trap as well.

The good news is that by eating the right foods we are able to help our bodies eliminate built up toxins and thus reduce inflammation. When you cut out the toxins your body has the chance to heal.

***Foods that contribute to inflammation*** include processed carbohydrates and sugars, which are the worst offenders. These are extremely low in nutrient content and are actually *anti-nutrient* foods, meaning in order to process them we are expending more energy than the foods are providing for us. Here is a basic list of some common pro-inflammatory foods:

- Refined carbohydrates (gluten, flour, cookies, cakes, crackers, bread, pasta, cereals)
- Processed soy
- A diet heavy in grains and legumes can be inflammatory for some. Grains and legumes should not be the base of your diet.
- Refined & Artificial Sweeteners: Stick to small amounts of raw honey and pure maple syrup if you need something sweet.
- Hydrogenated Fats & Oils: Eliminate anything labeled as hydrogenated or partially hydrogenated. You will also want to skip vegetable oils, and margarine. Coconut oil is a great option for cooking as it's very heat stable and does not oxidize as easily in the pan as some of the other oils.
- Non-organic dairy products
- Soda
- Excessive amounts of alcohol and caffeine
- Corn & other GMO products

*Seem overwhelming? Just think of all the* **foods you CAN enjoy!**

- Organic fruits and vegetables.
- Organic grass-fed animal products & wild caught fish
- Healthy Fats: Coconut, avocados, nuts, seeds, ghee, wild caught salmon, flax seeds, chia seeds.
- Herbs & Spices: Turmeric, ginger, garlic

# Why is an Anti-Inflammatory Diet Good For Your Health?

An anti-inflammatory diet is excellent for your health for a number of reasons. I have listed out the top 3 ways that an anti-inflammatory diet can be beneficial to your health below.

- **Eliminating Processed Foods:** When you are following an anti-inflammatory diet, you are eliminating processed foods from your diet. When you remove toxic processed foods from your diet you are also eliminating damaged fats such as trans fats and hydrogenated fats. You are eliminating artificial colors and additives from your diet as well as reducing refined flours and sodium content from your diet. When you eliminate all of these things you give your body the chance to naturally detoxify itself, which also reduces blood pressure and cholesterol levels. You may even see that it is much easier to lose weight and keep it off. Most importantly, you are reducing inflammation. When you reduce the inflammation in your body, you allow your body to heal in all other aspects as well.

- **Boosting Antioxidants:** Anti-inflammatory diets are full of antioxidant rich foods, such as berries, dark leafy greens and citrus fruits, which play a huge role in reducing inflammation, as well as supporting the immune system and eliminating free radicals. Free radicals are atoms or molecules that are missing an electron, which make them highly reactive. Through the process of oxidation, they take electrons from components of our cells, thereby causing damage to DNA, proteins, and other parts of our cells. Free radicals in the body are responsible for destroying healthy cells and they lead to degenerative diseases and premature aging. It is thought that free radicals come from many different substances, including UV rays, X-rays, pesticides, tobacco smoke, alcohol, fried foods and air pollutants. Dr. Denham Harman proposed this theory on free radicals back in 1954. His theory was ignored until the 1960s, when other scientists proved his theory right. His theory makes a whole lot of sense when it comes to what free radicals are doing to our body. The theory basically stated that all of the symptoms we normally associate with aging, as well as every disease there is, are caused by damage caused by free radicals on your body. These symptoms include decreased mental and motor function, pains and wrinkles, as well as Alzheimer's disease, arthritis and heart disease, which can all be linked to free radical damage in the body. This theory on free radicals stated that the location of the free radical damage determined the likely disease to follow. This makes a lot of sense when you think about lung disease and smokers. Smokers are more likely to get lung disease because of cigarette smoke damaging their lungs and causing free radicals (4). This is where the antioxidants come in. The antioxidants seen in the anti-inflammatory diet can combat the free radicals and give the body what it needs in order to fight against the damage that the free radicals cause. We need to have more antioxidants than free radicals in our body in order to prevent disease.

- **Creates an Alkaline Body:** The alkaline versus acidic state in our body is extremely important. We always want our bodies to be more alkaline than we do acidic. When our bodies are acidic, we will experience unwanted symptoms such as digestive distress, lack of energy, aches and pains, and inflammation. An alkaline body will allow you to have an improvement in energy, reduced amounts of joint pain, improved digestion and an overall sense of wellbeing. Foods that you find when following an anti-inflammatory diet such as omega-3 fatty acids, fruits and vegetables, clean proteins, and herbs and spices will also promote alkalinity in the body. Removing processed foods and toxins such as smoking, drinking alcohol, and excessive caffeine will also help to bring your body to a more alkaline state and reduce the amount of acidity in the body.

# Is an Anti-Inflammatory Diet a Good Way to Detox?

When we shift our diet away from pro-inflammatory and towards anti-inflammatory foods, we are, by default, detoxifying all body systems. If you have chosen to commit to making lasting changes, you are ready to get off the blood sugar rollercoaster and locate foods that you may be sensitive or allergic to and that may be compromising how you feel on a day-to-day basis.

Each individual may have a different motivation for wanting to take on an anti-inflammatory diet, and that is exactly how it should be. The beauty of an anti-inflammatory diet is that it will be beneficial to all, no matter your particular reasons.

Here are several reasons you may want to adopt an anti-inflammatory diet:

- You crave carbohydrates
- You feel like you always have to grab something sugary or have a dessert every night
- You are experiencing chronic fatigue
- You struggle with sleep
- You are constantly under stress
- You have frequent digestive complaints
- You suffer from allergies
- You feel like you have brain fog
- You experience frequent irritability
- You are frequently sick
- You struggle to lose weight
- You have frequent headaches
- You suffer from joint pain

This list is not all inclusive as you may experience other symptoms not on this list than relate back to inflammation. However, one of the many great things about changing your diet for the better and leaning more towards an anti-inflammatory diet is that it's safe and yet effective. By removing toxic foods from your diet, you not only support health but you can protect your health for the long term.

## Getting Over a Sugar Addiction

When you first start an anti-inflammatory diet, you may be surprised at your desire to consume sugar! If this is the case, you are not alone. Many of us struggle with a sugar dependence and it's no necessarily our fault, especially if we haven't been made aware of all of the hidden sources of sugar in our food. However, that stops now! You are now well equipped with the information you need to know about the foods that cause inflammation and that sugar is one of the top offenders. So, how do we break the sugar addiction?

First you need to understand why these cravings happen in the first place. Carbohydrates trigger the release of serotonin in the brain which is known to help us feel good. When we eat sugar, we experience that "sugar high" and it makes us want more. Sugar also tastes good and it can become very easy for us to get into the habit of rewarding ourselves with a sweet treat to experience those feel-good chemicals but the problem is that it soon becomes a sugar addiction. Americans consume an average of 22 teaspoons of added sugar per day according to the American Heart Association (5). That is an excessive amount of sugar and certainly something that can lead to inflammation.

By starting an anti-inflammatory diet, you will naturally be able to better regulate your blood sugar levels, as you will be meeting your body's nutritional needs and you will feel more satisfied after a meal as opposed to craving something sweet. Your body will eventually adjust and you will no longer have those strong sugar cravings, but these cravings are inevitable at the start.

Here are a few tips to help you get over that sugar craving hump:

- Get out of the kitchen and go for a brisk walk when those cravings kick in
- Call a friend or take a cat nap when you feel like you can't say no to sugar
- Snack on something that contains a decent amount of healthy fat such as nuts and seeds or an avocado
- Eat regular nourishing meals to keep your blood sugar levels stable
- If you're craving dessert, have a piece of fruit. Fruit is high in sugar to satisfy that craving but also comes with some anti-inflammatory benefits and some fiber.

## What Sugars You Should be Keeping Out of Your Diet:

- Aspartame
- Saccharin

- Sucralose
- High fructose corn syrup

**Natural Sweeteners to Use on Occasion:**

- Pure maple syrup
- Raw honey
- Molasses
- Freshly squeezed fruit juice
- Green leaf stevia (i.e. totally natural and unaltered stevia plant powder)

**Looking at Food Labels:**

- Focus on carbohydrate and sugar in grams: 4 grams of sugar = 1 tsp.
- Look out for ingredients ending in "ose" or "tol" (e.g.: sucralose, sucrose, fructose, sorbitol, xylitol)
- Avoid ingredients such as sugar, nectar, syrup, or crystals.
- Bear in mind that the ingredients are listed in terms of what percentage they are present in the food and the largest percentage is the first item listed.

You now know all about inflammation and you have the information you need to put an anti-inflammatory diet into action! Let's learn how to put this information into practice day-to-day with simple and delicious recipes.

# How to Get Started on an Anti-Inflammatory Diet?

If you are ready to start eating to promote health and fight inflammation, I am going to help guide you on how to get started on an anti-inflammatory diet. Changing the way you eat can be stressful and takes some planning. I am here to make the process stress-free and easy to follow. Starting on an anti-inflammatory diet is a commitment to a major lifestyle change. Anti-inflammatory diets are not so much diets as they are a lifestyle change. Changing the way you eat to combat inflammation and disease should be a lifelong change to help you live a long and healthy life.

1. **Start by reducing the amount of unhealthy fats in your diet:** Damaged fats and oils are super inflammatory. The 1st step in going anti-inflammatory is to remove these damaged fats from your diet. Swap out unhealthy oils for olive oil, avocado oil, and coconut oil, and enjoy more omega-3 rich foods instead of omega-6. Add in things like wild-caught salmon, walnuts, and flax seeds. Remove the margarine from your fridge as well.

2. **Focus on what you can have versus what you can't**: If you start to focus on all of the things that you have to remove from your diet, it takes you down a negative road. Think about all the healthy foods that you can enjoy and start to make a list.

3. **Take a look at Dr. Weil's anti-inflammatory food pyramid:** Start to make a list of all of the foods you know you will enjoy on Dr. Weil's food pyramid, and follow how many serving you are allowed to have per day. *Note: Refer to Dr. Weil's website for anti-inflammatory food pyramid.*

4. **Remember that not all of life's fun foods are off the table:** Eating anti-inflammatory foods does not mean you will never be able to indulge again. You may have noticed on Dr. Weil's pyramid that dark chocolate and red wine are listed, just in moderation. Life is about moderation. You can still enjoy those occasional treats, and knowing this makes following any kind of diet much easier.

# Do's & Don't on an Anti-Inflammatory Diet

**Do's of the Anti-Inflammatory Diet:**

- Do get your omega-3 fatty acids in.
- Do enjoy dark chocolate and red wine from time to time. Just be sure the chocolate is at least 70% dark cocoa and unsweetened
- Do enjoy healthy fats such as olive oil, coconut oil, nuts, seeds, and avocados.
- Do get plenty of rest.
- Do get plenty of exercise in your day.
- Do manage stress levels.

**Dont's of the Anti-Inflammatory Diet:**

- Don't eat processed junk foods.
- Don't consume damaged oils
- Don't smoke or put any toxins into your body.
- Don't use toxic household cleaners.
- Don't consume processed and artificial sweeteners.
- Don't overdo the caffeine or alcohol.

# What Foods Are Best to Fight Inflammation & What Foods Cause Inflammation

Now that we have an understanding as to what an anti-inflammatory diet is, and how it can benefit our health. Let's take a look at some of the foods that are best at fighting inflammation, as well as the foods that you are going to want to completely eliminate your diet on an anti-inflammatory diet.

**Foods That Fight Inflammation**

**These foods should be enjoyed often:**

- Leafy greens
- Vegetables
- Fruits
- Raw nut butters
- Herbal tea
- Herbs and spices: turmeric, ginger, cinnamon
- Green tea
- Wild-caught salmon
- Anchovies
- Sardines
- Avocados
- Sprouts
- Coconut kefir
- Raw nuts and seeds
- Extra virgin olive oil
- Green juices and smoothies
- Organic Pasture raised eggs
- Soaked and sprouted grains
- Seaweed
- Apple cider vinegar
- Squash
- Sweet potatoes

**Please note that this is not an exclusive list.**

# Foods That Promote Inflammation

**These foods should be avoided:**

- Processed and commercial meats
- Dairy products except for high-quality cheeses in moderation
- Alcohol
- Nicotine
- Refined grains
- Processed soy
- Processed and artificial sugars
- Highly processed foods (cereals, chips, packages snacks)
- Caffeine (except green tea)
- Fried foods
- Fast foods
- Sodas
- Energy drinks

# Food Groups

**Dr. Weil's Recommendations (6)**

**Carbohydrates:**

- These carbohydrates should be from unrefined sources – whole grains, such as brown rice.
- Other carbohydrates such as beans, squash and sweet potatoes may also be consumed.
- If consuming pasta, try brown rice pasta and cook to al dente.

**Fats:**

- Reduce your intake of saturated fats by reducing the amount of butter, cream, high fat cheese, unskinned chicken and fatty meats.
- Use extra virgin olive oil as your primary oil.
- Avoid safflower oil, corn oil, cottonseed oil, vegetable oils, margarine, and vegetable shortening.
- Enjoy omega-3 rich foods choose options such as wild caught salmon, sardines, herring, organic, and pasture raised eggs, hemp seeds, and flax seeds.

**Proteins:**

- Try to decrease the amount of animal protein you eat except for fish.
- Eat more plant based proteins such as beans.

**Fiber:**

- Women should strive for 25 grams of fiber per day while men need about 38 grams per day according to the Institute of Medicine (7).
- Foods high in fiber include berries, vegetables and whole grains.

# BREAKFAST RECIPES

# Berry Coconut Porridge

**Preparation time:** 5 minutes
**Cooking time:** 10 minutes
**Makes:** 3 servings

## Ingredients:

- 1 and a ½ cups of gluten-free rolled oats
- 2 tablespoons of chia seeds
- 3 cups of almond milk
- 2 tablespoons of raw cocoa nibs
- 2 tablespoons of shredded coconut
- 1 cup of blueberries (frozen or fresh)

## Directions:

1. Start by cooking the rolled oats with the almond milk and chia seeds over medium heat, and simmer until the oats are cooked.

2. Pour into three serving bowls and top with shredded coconut, raw cocoa nibs and berries.

3. Serve warm.

## Nutrition Facts (per serving)

Total Carbohydrates: 56g
Dietary Fiber: 15g
Protein: 11g
Total Fat: 18g
Calories: 416

# Anti-Inflammatory Berry Smoothie

**Preparation time:** 10 minutes
**Cooking time:** 0 minutes
**Makes:** 2 servings

## Ingredients:

½ cup of raspberries
½ cup of blueberries
½ frozen banana
1 cup of dairy-free unsweetened milk
1 tablespoon of flaxseeds
1 handful of fresh spinach
1 tablespoon of almond butter

## Directions:

1. Place all ingredients into a high speed blender, and blend until smooth.

2. Drink immediately or store in the fridge for later.

## Nutrition Facts (per serving)

Total Carbohydrates: 26g
Dietary Fiber: 8g
Protein: 4g
Total Fat: 9g
Calories: 185

# Gingerbread Buckwheat Cereal

**Preparation time:** 5 minutes
**Cooking time:** 3 minutes
**Makes:** 3 servings

## Ingredients:

1 cup of buckwheat groats
1 and a ½ cups of full-fat canned coconut milk
½ teaspoon of ground ginger
1 teaspoon of ground cinnamon
1 tablespoon of raw cocoa powder
2 tablespoons of pumpkin seeds
2 tablespoons of pure maple syrup

## Directions:

1. Place the buckwheat groats and coconut milk in a medium pot over medium heat, and add in the ginger, cinnamon and raw cocoa. Stir.

2. Bring this to a boil, and let it simmer until the buckwheat groats are cooked (about 2-3 minutes).

3. Pour into three serving bowls, and top with a tablespoon of pumpkin seeds and a tablespoon of pure maple syrup per serving.

## Nutrition Facts (per serving)

Total Carbohydrates: 487g
Dietary Fiber: 8g
Protein: 10g
Total Fat: 31g
Calories: 487

# Gluten-Free Crepes

**Preparation time:** 10 minutes
**Cooking time:** 4 minutes
**Makes:** 6 servings

## Ingredients:

2 organic pasture-raised eggs
1 teaspoon of pure vanilla extract
½ cup of unsweetened almond milk
½ cup of water
¼ teaspoon of salt

1 tablespoon of pure maple syrup
1 cup of gluten-free all-purpose flour
2 tablespoons of coconut oil, melted
1 tablespoon of coconut oil for cooking

### *Filling Options:*

Strawberries, blueberries and honey.
Nut butter with bananas.

## Directions:

1. Place 2 tablespoons of coconut oil into a small saucepan, and melt over low heat. Set aside.

2. Whisk the eggs, vanilla, unsweetened nut milk, water, salt and pure maple syrup together in a mixing bowl.

3. Next, add in the flour and whisk to combine.

4. Add the melted oil to the batter and whisk to combine.

5. Heat a teaspoon of coconut oil in a large frying pan over medium high heat.

6. Pour a third of a cup of the batter onto the frying pan, and quickly tilt and swirl the pan in a circular motion so that the batter coats the surface evenly.

7. Cook each crepe for 2 minutes, being careful not to burn the bottom.

8. Flip, and cook the other side for 2 minutes.

9. Cook each crepe in this manner.

10. Once the crepes are all cooked, add your fillings of choice: berries with honey or nut butter with bananas.

**Nutrition Facts (per serving, without fillings)**

Total Carbohydrates: 14g
Dietary Fiber: 1g
Protein: 4g
Total Fat: 8g
Calories: 143

# Veggie Omelet

**Preparation time:** 5 minutes
**Cooking time:** 10 minutes
**Makes:** 1 serving

## Ingredients:

2 organic pasture-raised eggs
½ teaspoon of turmeric
1 handful of fresh spinach
¼ cup of mushrooms
2 tablespoons of chopped onion
Himalayan sea salt to taste
1 tablespoon of coconut oil for cooking

## Directions:

1. Whisk the eggs together with the turmeric. Add in the mushrooms, onions and fresh spinach.

2. Heat a tablespoon of coconut oil in a small frying pan over medium heat.

3. Add the egg mixture to the pan, and cook for about 5 minutes.

4. Flip 1 side of the omelet on top of the other, and let this cook for another 2 minutes. Flip and cook for 2 more minutes.

5. Serve with Himalayan sea salt to taste.

## Nutrition Facts (per serving)

Total Carbohydrates: 5g
Dietary Fiber: 1g
Protein: 13g
Total Fat: 22g
Calories: 266

# Avocado Eggs with Balsamic Vinegar

**Preparation time:** 5 minutes
**Cooking time:** 5 minutes
**Makes:** 1 serving

## Ingredients:

2 organic pasture-raised eggs
½ avocado
1 slice of tomato
1 tablespoon of balsamic vinegar

## Directions:

1. Start by frying the eggs to your liking, whilst peeling and slicing the avocado.

2. Place the avocado on a plate, and top with the cooked eggs, sliced tomato and a drizzle of balsamic vinegar.

## Nutrition Facts (per serving)

Total Carbohydrates: 10g
Dietary Fiber: 5g
Protein: 13g
Total Fat: 19g
Calories: 252

# Ginger Turmeric Shake

**Preparation time:** 5 minutes
**Cooking time:** 0 minutes
**Makes:** 1 serving

## Ingredients:

1 blood orange
½ cup of frozen mango
1/3 cup of coconut water
½ teaspoon of ground ginger
1 teaspoon of ground turmeric
½ teaspoon of ground cinnamon
1 pinch of cayenne pepper

## Directions:

1. Place all ingredients into a high speed blender, and blend until smooth.

2. Pour into a glass, and enjoy straight away.

## Nutrition Facts (per serving)

Total Carbohydrates: 34g
Dietary Fiber: 6g
Protein: 3g
Total Fat: 1g
Calories: 138

# Dairy-Free Antioxidant Yogurt Parfait

**Preparation time:** 5minutes
**Cooking time:** 0 minutes
**Makes:** 2 servings

## Ingredients:

- 1 cup of full-fat, unsweetened coconut yogurt
- 1 cup of wild blueberries
- 2 tablespoons of ground flaxseeds
- 2 tablespoons of hemp seeds
- 2 tablespoons of chopped walnuts
- 2 teaspoons of raw honey

## Directions:

1. Divide the coconut milk yogurt between two serving bowls or cups.

2. Top the yogurt with half a cup of wild berries per serving, with 1 tablespoon of ground flax seeds, 1 tablespoon hemp seeds, 1 tablespoon of chopped walnuts and 1 teaspoon of raw honey each.

## Nutrition Facts (per serving)

Total Carbohydrates: 28g
Dietary Fiber: 7g
Protein: 9g
Total Fat: 16g
Calories: 275

# Power Pancakes

**Preparation time:** 15 minutes
**Cooking time:** 25 minutes
**Makes:** 6 servings

## Ingredients:

4 organic pasture-raised eggs
1/4 cup of organic orange juice
1 ¼ cup of organic unsweetened almond milk
2 cups of gluten free white rice flour
1 teaspoon of aluminum-free baking powder

Coconut oil for cooking

*Toppings:*

1 and a ½ cups of sliced bananas
6 tablespoons of crushed walnuts
1 and a ½ cups of pure maple syrup

## Directions:

1. Whisk the eggs, and add in the orange juice and almond milk. Be careful not to over whisk.

2. Combine all of the dry ingredients together in a separate mixing bowl, and stir until combined.

3. Gradually stir the dry ingredients into the wet ingredients, and mix until well combined.

4. Heat up a large skillet with 1 tablespoon of coconut oil. Pour 3 tablespoons of the batter onto the pan and cook 2 minutes each side. Transfer the pancake to a warm dish, and continue to cook each pancake this way.

5. Top with ¼ cup of sliced bananas, 1 tablespoon crushed walnuts and ¼ cup pure maple syrup per serving.

## Nutrition Facts (per serving)

Total Carbohydrates: 109g
Dietary Fiber: 3g
Protein: 8g
Total Fat: 8g
Calories: 538

# Anti-Inflammatory Muffins

**Preparation time:** 15 minutes
**Cooking time:** 25 minutes
**Makes:** 12 servings

## Ingredients:

2 cups of almond flour
½ teaspoon of sea salt
2 teaspoons of aluminum-free baking powder
4 organic pasture-raised eggs
2 ripe bananas, mashed

1 cup of organic canned sweet potatoes
¼ cup of olive oil
1 teaspoon of ground turmeric
1 teaspoon of ground ginger
1 teaspoon of ground cinnamon

## Directions:

1. Start by preheating the oven to 400°F and lining a muffin pan with 12 muffin liners.

2. Whisk the eggs and then mix in the olive oil.

3. Mash the bananas, and add to the egg mixture. Stir in the canned sweet potatoes.

4. Combine the almond flour, sea salt, baking powder and spices in a separate bowl and stir.

5. Gradually add the flour mixture to the wet ingredients, stirring all the time until smooth.

6. Divide the mixture between the muffin liners, and bake for 20 to 25 minutes or until a toothpick comes out clean

## Nutrition Facts (per serving)

Total Carbohydrates: 14g
Dietary Fiber: 4g
Protein: 7g
Total Fat: 18g
Calories: 235

# Matcha Smoothie Bowl

**Preparation time:** 10 minutes
**Cooking time:** 0 minutes
**Makes:** 2 servings

## Ingredients:

1 cup of canned coconut milk
1 cup of fresh spinach
1 cup of frozen mango
2 tablespoons of green tea matcha powder
2 tablespoons of pure maple syrup

*Toppings:*

1 tablespoon chia seeds
1 tablespoon shredded coconut

## Directions:

1. Place all of the ingredients, except for the toppings, into a high speed blender and blend until smooth.

2. Top with the chia seeds and shredded coconut.

## Nutrition Facts (per serving)

Total Carbohydrates: 39g
Dietary Fiber: 7g
Protein: 5g
Total Fat: 32g
Calories: 433

# Vanilla Berry Smoothie Bowl

**Preparation time:** 10 minutes
**Cooking time:** 0 minutes
**Makes:** 2 servings

## Ingredients:

1 frozen banana
1 cup of fresh spinach
1 cup of frozen blueberries
1 teaspoon of pure vanilla extract
2 tablespoons of pure maple syrup
¼ cup of unsweetened almond milk

## Directions:

1. Place all ingredients into a high speed blender and blend until smooth.

2. Pour into a glass, and enjoy straight away.

## Nutrition Facts (per serving)

Total Carbohydrates: 53g
Dietary Fiber: 5g
Protein: 2g
Total Fat: 1g
Calories: 210

# Orange Kefir Chia Pudding

**Preparation time:** 10 minutes
**Cooking time:** 1.5 hours
**Makes:** 1 serving

## Ingredients:

Juice of 1 orange
1 tablespoon of pure maple syrup
1 teaspoon of pure vanilla extract
1 tablespoon of chia seeds
½ cup of kefir

## Directions:

1. Place all of the ingredients into a mixing bowl, and whisk until combined.

2. Place in the refrigerator for 1 and a half hours, until the chia seeds have created a pudding-like texture.

3. Enjoy chilled.

## Nutrition Facts (per serving)

Total Carbohydrates: 38g
Dietary Fiber: 5g
Protein: 7g
Total Fat: 6g
Calories: 226

# Sweet Potato Toast

**Preparation time:** 15 minutes
**Cooking time:** 35 minutes
**Makes:** 1 serving

## Ingredients:

2 sweet potatoes
1 avocado, mashed
4 organic pasture-raised eggs, cooked to your liking over easy.
Sea salt to taste

## Directions:

1. Preheat the oven to 375°F.

2. Wash and cut the uncooked sweet potato into 4 thin strips.

3. Cook the sweet potato for about 35 minutes, or until thoroughly cooked.

4. Once the sweet potatoes are cooked, spread a quarter of the avocado on each piece, and top with a cooked egg each. Season with salt.

## Nutrition Facts (per serving)

Total Carbohydrates: 26g
Dietary Fiber: 8g
Protein: 14g
Total Fat: 19g
Calories: 317

# Inflammation-Busting Zucchini Muffins

**Preparation time:** 15 minutes
**Cooking time:** 30 minutes
**Makes:** 18 servings

## Ingredients:

1 and a ½ cups of almond flour
½ cup of rice flour
2 teaspoons of aluminum-free baking powder
1 teaspoon of ground cinnamon
1 teaspoon of ground nutmeg
½ cup of melted coconut oil
2 organic pasture-raised eggs
1 cup of shredded zucchini
½ cup of pure maple syrup

## Directions:

1. Start by preheating your oven to 350°F and lining a muffin pan with muffin liners.

2. Whisk together all of the dry ingredients, and then whisk in the eggs, pure maple syrup and melted coconut oil. Finally, whisk in the zucchini.

3. Fill each muffin liner about three quarters of the way full, and bake for 30 minutes, or until a toothpick comes out clean.

4. Serve with a smear of coconut oil.

## Nutrition Facts (per serving)

Total Carbohydrates: 12g
Dietary Fiber: 1g
Protein: 3g
Total Fat: 11g
Calories: 146

# LUNCH RECIPES

# Clean Eating Egg Salad

**Preparation time:** 10 minutes
**Cooking time:** 0 minutes
**Makes:** 2 servings

## Ingredients:

6 organic pasture-raised eggs, hard boiled
1 avocado
¼ cup of Greek yogurt
2 tablespoons of olive oil mayonnaise
1 teaspoon of fresh dill
Sea salt to taste
Lettuce for serving

## Directions:

1. Mash the hard boiled eggs and avocado together.

2. Add in the Greek yogurt, olive oil mayonnaise and fresh dill.

3. Season with sea salt.

4. Serve on a bed of lettuce.

## Nutrition Facts (per serving)

Total Carbohydrates: 18g
Dietary Fiber: 10g
Protein: 23g
Total Fat: 38g
Calories: 486

# Healthy Tuna Salad

**Preparation time:** 10 minutes
**Cooking time:** 0 minutes
**Makes:** 2 servings

## Ingredients:

1 (6.5 ounce) can of wild tuna packed in olive oil
1 apple
1 stalk of celery
2 tablespoons of olive oil mayonnaise
2 tablespoons of Greek yogurt
1 pinch of cayenne pepper

## Directions:

1. Start by chopping the apple and celery into cubes.

2. Combine the tuna, apple, celery, mayonnaise, Greek yogurt and cayenne pepper together.

3. Serve with a side of lettuce or fresh, raw vegetables.

## Nutrition Facts (per serving)

Total Carbohydrates: 13g
Dietary Fiber: 2g
Protein: 25g
Total Fat: 10g
Calories: 241

# Kale Caesar Salad Wraps

**Preparation time:** 10 minutes
**Cooking time:** 0 minutes
**Makes:** 2 servings

## Ingredients:

1 cup of grilled organic chicken, sliced
4 cups of kale, chopped into small pieces
1 cup of cherry tomatoes, sliced
1 cup of purple grapes, sliced in half
1 teaspoon of Dijon mustard
1 teaspoon of raw honey
1/8 cup of olive oil
2 (6 inch) gluten-free tortillas

## Directions:

1. In a small bowl, whisk together the Dijon mustard, honey, and olive oil to make the dressing.

2. Add the chicken, kale, tomatoes and grapes to the dressing bowl, and toss gently.

3. Divide the filling between the two tortillas.

4. Roll up into wraps, cut in half and enjoy right away.

## Nutrition Facts (per serving)

Total Carbohydrates: 45g
Dietary Fiber: 8g
Protein: 29g
Total Fat: 11g
Calories: 377

# Winter Style Fruit Salad

**Preparation time:** 10 minutes
**Cooking time:** 0 minutes
**Makes:** 6 servings

## Ingredients:

4 cooked sweet potatoes, cubed (1-inch cubes)
3 pears, cubed (1-inch cubes)
1 cup of grapes, halved
1 apple, cubed
½ cup of pecan halves
2 tablespoons of olive oil
1 tablespoon of red wine vinegar
2 tablespoons of raw honey

## Directions:

1. Start by whisking together the olive oil, red wine vinegar and raw honey to make the dressing, and set aside.

2. Combine the chopped fruit, sweet potato and pecan halves, and divide this between six serving bowls.

3. Drizzle each bowl with the dressing.

## Nutrition Facts (per serving)

Total Carbohydrates: 40g
Dietary Fiber: 6g
Protein: 3g
Total Fat: 11g
Calories: 251

# Easy Salmon Salad

**Preparation time:** 10 minutes
**Cooking time:** 0 minutes
**Makes:** 1 serving

## Ingredients:

1 cup of organic arugula
1 (6.5 ounce) can of wild-caught salmon
½ of an avocado, sliced
1 tablespoon of olive oil
1 teaspoon of Dijon mustard
1 teaspoon of sea salt

## Directions:

1. Start by whisking the olive oil, Dijon mustard and sea salt together in a mixing bowl to make the dressing. Set aside.

2. Assemble the salad with the arugula as the base, and top with the salmon and sliced avocado.

3. Drizzle with the dressing.

## Nutrition Facts (per serving)

Total Carbohydrates: 7g
Dietary Fiber: 5g
Protein: 48g
Total Fat: 37g
Calories: 553

# Quinoa Salad

**Preparation time:** 15 minutes
**Cooking time:** 20 minutes
**Makes:** 4 servings

## Ingredients:

1 cup of uncooked quinoa, rinsed
½ a red onion, chopped
1 apple, chopped
2 tablespoons of raw honey
1 tablespoon of olive oil
1 large mango, chopped
1 teaspoon of ground ginger
1 avocado, chopped
1 cup of cashews, chopped
3 cups of kale, chopped

## Directions:

1. Cook the quinoa in 2 cups of boiling water for 20 minutes. Set aside.

2. Put the chopped onion and apple in a mixing bowl. Add the honey and olive oil and mix well.

3. Stir in the cooked quinoa, mango and ginger.

4. Garnish the quinoa salad with chopped avocado and chopped cashews.

5. Scoop the salad over a bed of kale.

6. Best if served chilled.

## Nutrition Facts (per serving)

Total Carbohydrates: 64g
Dietary Fiber: 9g
Protein: 13g
Total Fat: 23g
Calories: 491

# Healthy Pasta Salad

**Preparation time:** 15 minutes
**Cooking time:** 10 minutes
**Makes:** 6 servings

## Ingredients:

1 package of gluten-free fusilli pasta
1 cup of grape tomatoes, sliced
1 handful of fresh cilantro, chopped
1 cup of olives, halved
1 cup of fresh basil, chopped
½ cup of olive oil
Sea salt to taste

## Directions:

1. Whisk together the olive oil, chopped basil, cilantro and sea salt. Set aside.

2. Cook the pasta according to package directions, strain, and rinse.

3. Combine the pasta with the tomatoes and olives.

4. Add the olive oil mixture, and toss until well combined.

## Nutrition Facts (per serving)

Total Carbohydrates: 66g
Dietary Fiber: 5g
Protein: 13g
Total Fat: 23g
Calories: 525

# Spinach Bean Salad

**Preparation time:** 10 minutes
**Cooking time:** 5 minutes
**Makes:** 1 serving

## Ingredients:

1 cup of fresh spinach
¼ cup of canned black beans
½ cup of canned garbanzo beans
½ cup of cremini mushrooms
2 tablespoons of organic balsamic vinaigrette
1 tablespoon of olive oil

## Directions:

1. Cook the cremini mushrooms with the olive oil over a low medium heat for 5 minutes, until lightly browned.

2. Assemble the salad by adding the fresh spinach to a plate, and topping it with the beans, mushrooms, and the balsamic vinaigrette.

## Nutrition Facts (per serving)

Total Carbohydrates: 26gg
Dietary Fiber: 8g
Protein: 9g
Total Fat: 15g
Calories: 274

# Anti-Inflammatory Kale Salad

**Preparation time:** 10 minutes
**Cooking time:** 0 minutes
**Makes:** 1 serving

## Ingredients:

1 cup of fresh kale
½ cup of blueberries
½ cup of pitted cherries, halved
¼ cup of dried cranberries
1 tablespoon of sesame seeds
2 tablespoons of olive oil
Juice of 1 lemon

## Directions:

1. Start by whisking together the olive oil and lemon juice, and then toss the kale in the dressing.

2. Place the kale leaves into a large salad bowl, and top with the fresh blueberries, cherries and cranberries.

3. Top with the sesame seeds.

## Nutrition Facts (per serving)

Total Carbohydrates: 48g
Dietary Fiber: 7g
Protein: 6g
Total Fat: 33g
Calories: 477

# Sweet Potato Soup

**Preparation time:** 15 minutes
**Cooking time:** 15 minutes
**Makes:** 6 servings

## Ingredients:

2 tablespoons of olive oil
1 medium onion, chopped
1 (4 ounce) can of green chilies
1 teaspoon of ground cumin
1 teaspoon of ground ginger
1 teaspoon of sea salt
4 cups of sweet potatoes, peeled and chopped
4 cups of organic, low-sodium vegetable broth
2 tablespoons of fresh cilantro, minced
6 tablespoons of Greek yogurt

## Directions:

1. In a large soup pot, heat the olive oil over medium heat. Add in the onion, and sauté until soft. Add in the green chilies and seasonings, and cook for 2 minutes.

2. Stir in the sweet potatoes and vegetable broth, and bring to a boil.

3. Simmer for 15 minutes, or until the sweet potatoes are tender.

4. Stir in the minced cilantro.

5. Place half of the soup into a blender or food processor, and blend until smooth. Add back to the pot with the remaining soup.

6. Season with extra sea salt if desired, and top with a dollop of Greek yogurt.

## Nutrition Facts (per serving)

Total Carbohydrates: 33g
Dietary Fiber: 5g
Protein: 6g
Total Fat: 5g
Calories: 192

# Curry Lentil Stew

**Preparation time:** 10 minutes
**Cooking time:** 15 minutes
**Makes:** 4 servings

## Ingredients:

1 tablespoon of olive oil
1 onion, chopped
2 garlic cloves, minced
1 tablespoon of organic curry seasoning
4 cups of organic low-sodium vegetable broth
1 cup of red lentils
2 cups of butternut squash, cooked
1 cup of kale
1 teaspoon of turmeric
Sea salt to taste

## Directions:

1. In a large pot over medium heat, add the olive oil with the onion and garlic. Sauté for 3 minutes.

2. Add in the organic curry seasoning, vegetable broth and lentils, and bring to a boil. Cook for 10 minutes.

3. Stir in the cooked butternut squash and kale.

4. Add in the turmeric and sea salt to taste.

5. Serve warm.

## Nutrition Facts (per serving)

Total Carbohydrates: 41g
Dietary Fiber: 13g
Protein: 16g
Total Fat: 4g
Calories: 252

# Black Bean Tortilla Wrap

**Preparation time:** 10 minutes
**Cooking time:** 0 minutes
**Makes:** 2 servings

## Ingredients:

¼ cup of corn
1 handful of fresh basil
½ cup of arugula
1 tablespoon of nutritional yeast
¼ cup of canned black beans
1 peach, sliced
1 teaspoon of lime juice
2 (8 inch) gluten-free tortillas

## Directions:

1.  Divide the beans, corn, arugula and peaches between the two tortillas.

2.  Top each tortilla with half the fresh basil and lime juice

## Nutrition Facts (per serving)

Total Carbohydrates: 44g
Dietary Fiber: 7g
Protein: 8g
Total Fat: 1g
Calories: 203

# Sweet Potato Patties

**Preparation time:** 10 minutes
**Cooking time:** 5 minutes
**Makes:** 4 servings

## Ingredients:

2 ½ cups of sweet potato, peeled & shredded
1/3 cup of rice flour
½ cup of white onion, chopped
1 large organic pasture-raised egg, beaten
12 tablespoons coconut oil for cooking
Salt and pepper to taste

## Directions:

1. Combine the sweet potato and flour in a large mixing bowl, and stir until the sweet potato is evenly coated. Add the onion and egg, and mix all together.

2. Divide the sweet potato mixture into four balls and form each one into a small patty.

3. Add 12 tablespoons of coconut oil to a pan over medium heat and allow to melt,

4. Cook each patty for 3 minutes, or until they are golden brown, on each side.

5. Serve with a side salad for the perfect anti-inflammatory lunch.

## Nutrition Facts (per serving)

Total Carbohydrates: 72g
Dietary Fiber: 10g
Protein: 8g
Total Fat: 5g
Calories: 359

# Coconut Mushroom Soup

**Preparation time:** 10 minutes
**Cooking time:** 10 minutes
**Makes:** 3 servings

## Ingredients:

1 tablespoon of coconut oil
1 tablespoon of ground ginger
1 cup of cremini mushrooms, chopped
½ teaspoon of turmeric
2 and a ½ cups of water
½ cup canned coconut milk
Sea salt to taste

## Directions:

1. Heat the coconut oil over medium heat in a large pot, and add the mushrooms. Cook for 3-4 minutes.

2. Add the remaining ingredients and bring to a low boil. Let it simmer for 5 minutes.

3. Divide between three soup bowls, and enjoy!

## Nutrition Facts (per serving)

Total Carbohydrates: 4g
Dietary Fiber: 1g
Protein: 2g
Total Fat: 14g
Calories: 143

# Tomato Detox Soup

**Preparation time:** 10 minutes
**Cooking time:** 20 minutes
**Makes:** 2 servings

## Ingredients:

½ cup of organic, low-sodium vegetable stock
1 (14.5 ounce) can of diced organic tomatoes
2 teaspoons of turmeric
1 teaspoon of olive oil
2 cloves of garlic
1 small onion, chopped
1 handful of fresh basil

## Directions:

1. Place all of the ingredients into a large stock pot, and bring to a boil.

2. Simmer for 20 minutes.

3. With an immersion blender, blend until smooth.

4. Serve with a slice of gluten-free toast or a side salad

## Nutrition Facts (per serving)

Total Carbohydrates: 14g
Dietary Fiber: 5g
Protein: 3g
Total Fat: 3g
Calories: 86

# Cauliflower Soup

**Preparation time:** 5 minutes
**Cooking time:** 10 minutes
**Makes:** 10 servings

## Ingredients:

¾ cup of water
2 teaspoon of olive oil
1 onion, diced
1 head of cauliflower, only the florets
1 can of full fat coconut milk
1 teaspoon of turmeric
1 teaspoon of ginger
1 teaspoon raw honey

## Directions:

1. Place all of the ingredients into a large stock pot, and boil for about 10 minutes.

2. Use an immersion blender to blend, and make the soup smooth. If you are using a blender, let the soup cool before blending.

## Nutrition Facts (per serving)

Total Carbohydrates: 7g
Dietary Fiber: 2g
Net Carbs:
Protein: 2g
Total Fat: 11g
Calories: 129

# DINNER RECIPES

# Fettuccine with Superfood Pesto

**Preparation time:** 20 minutes
**Cooking time:** 10 minutes
**Makes:** 6 servings

## Ingredients:

1 package of gluten-free fettuccine
½ cup of feta cheese, cubed
Pesto
1 cup of chopped kale
1 cup of basil
½ cup of olive oil
¼ cup of pine nuts
2 cloves of garlic
Salt and pepper to taste

## Directions:

1. Start by bringing a large pot of water to a boil, and cook the gluten-free fettuccine according to the package direction.

2. While the spaghetti is cooking, blend all the ingredients for the pesto in a high speed blender until smooth. Set aside.

3. Drain and rinse the pasta, and return it to the pot. Add in the pesto and feta, and stir.

4. Serve right away!

## Nutrition Facts (per serving)

Total Carbohydrates: 50g
Dietary Fiber: 3g
Protein: 12g
Total Fat: 3g
Calories: 480

# Baked Tilapia

**Preparation time:** 20 minutes
**Cooking time:** 10 minutes
**Makes:** 4 servings

## Ingredients:

½ cup of raw pecans, chopped
¼ cup of almond meal
2 teaspoons of fresh rosemary, chopped
⅛ teaspoon of salt
1 pinch of cayenne pepper
1 and a ½ teaspoons of olive oil
1 egg white
4 tilapia fillets (4 ounces each)

## Directions:

1. Preheat oven to 400°F.

2. In a mixing bowl, stir together pecans, almond meal, salt and cayenne pepper. Mix in 1 tsp. of the olive oil.

3. Coat a large glass baking dish with the remaining ½ tsp. of olive oil.

4. In a shallow dish, whisk the egg white. Working with one tilapia fillet at a time, dip the fish in the egg white and then the pecan mixture, lightly coating each side.

5. Place the fillets in the prepared baking dish.

6. Bake for 10 minutes, or until the tilapia is cooked through.

## Nutrition Facts (per serving)

Total Carbohydrates: 4g
Dietary Fiber: 2g
Protein: 26g
Total Fat: 19g
Calories: 276

# Tomato & Avocado Salad

**Preparation time:** 10 minutes
**Cooking time:** 0 minutes
**Makes:** 1 serving

## Ingredients:

1 cup of arugula
1 tomato, sliced
½ of an avocado, sliced
½ cup of canned chickpeas
½ teaspoon of black pepper
1 tablespoon of olive oil
2 tablespoons of balsamic vinegar
2 tablespoons of nutritional yeast

## Directions:

1. Assemble your salad with the arugula as a base, followed by the tomato slices, the avocado slices and then the chickpeas.

2. Sprinkle with the black pepper.

3. Mix the olive oil and balsamic vinegar and drizzle over the salad.

4. Sprinkle with nutritional yeast.

## Nutrition Facts (per serving)

Total Carbohydrates: 28g
Dietary Fiber: 10g
Protein: 7g
Total Fat: 25g
Calories: 356

# Superfood Bowl

**Preparation time:** 30 minutes
**Cooking time:** 40 minutes
**Makes:** 2 servings

## Ingredients:

¼ cup of uncooked quinoa, rinsed
½ a sweet potato, peeled & cubed
½ cup of lentils
¼ of an avocado
2 large stalks of kale
½ cup of cauliflower
½ cup of canned black beans
1 tablespoon of tahini dressing
Himalayan sea salt to taste

## Directions:

1. Start by baking the sweet potato at 375°F for 25 minutes, turning halfway through.

2. While the potatoes are cooking, rinse the quinoa and bring a quarter of a cup of dry quinoa to a boil with half a cup of water. Simmer for 20 minutes, adding more water if needed.

3. Rinse and cook the lentils by bringing 1 cup of water to a boil. Boil the lentils for 25 minutes.

4. Sauté the kale, steam the cauliflower and slice the avocado.

5. Place your cooked quinoa into a serving bowl, and top with all of the vegetables and lentils.

6. Drizzle with tahini, and add salt to taste.

## Nutrition Facts (per serving)

Total Carbohydrates: 60gg
Dietary Fiber: 19g
Protein: 21g
Total Fat: 9g
Calories: 386

# Red Salmon Cabbage Salad

**Preparation time:** 15 minutes
**Cooking time:** 10 minutes
**Makes:** 2 serving

## Ingredients:

1 cup of red cabbage, chopped
1 cucumber, sliced
1 tablespoon of mango salsa
1 tablespoon of almond butter
½ cup of cooked quinoa
1 (6.5 ounce) can of wild-caught salmon

## Directions:

1. Start by whisking the mango salsa, and almond butter together to make the dressing and set it aside.

2. Sauté the canned salmon over a medium heat for about 7 minutes, until browned.

3. Mix the red cabbage, and sliced cucumber together.

4. Place the salmon on top and then drizzle with the dressing.

5. Serve with the cooked quinoa on the side.

## Nutrition Facts (per serving)

Total Carbohydrates: 21g
Dietary Fiber: 4g
Protein: 24g
Total Fat: 16g
Calories: 324

# Black Bean Burgers

**Preparation time:** 10 minutes
**Cooking time:** 20 minutes
**Makes:** 4 servings

## Ingredients:

1 (15.5oz.) can of black beans
1/2 of a yellow onion, minced
½ of a jalapeno pepper, minced
2 cloves of garlic, minced
½ cup of brown rice, cooked
¼ teaspoon of red pepper flakes
Spice blend to your taste: Cayenne, cumin, pepper, salt

## Directions:

1. Preheat oven to 350 degrees Fahrenheit, and line a baking tray with parchment paper.

2. Drain and rinse the black beans.

3. With a potato masher, mash the black beans and rice.

4. Add the remaining ingredients and mix well.

5. Take a small handful of the mixture and roll into a ball. Continue to make small balls from the mixture until it is all used up.

6. Press each ball gently down onto the baking tray to make a burger shape.

7. Cook for 10 minutes and then turn the burgers over and cook for another 10 minutes.

8. Serve with some salad and/or a gluten-free wrap. (Not included in nutritional information)

## Nutrition Facts (per serving)

Total Carbohydrates: 34g
Dietary Fiber: 10g
Protein: 10g
Total Fat: 1g
Calories: 177

# Shrimp Quinoa Stir Fry

**Preparation time:** 15 minutes
**Cooking time:** 20 minutes
**Makes:** 4 servings

## Ingredients:

1 cup of uncooked quinoa, rinsed
1 and a ½ cups of water
1 pound of shrimp
1 clove of garlic
1 large head of broccoli, chopped
4 teaspoons of coconut oil
½ (24 ounce) jar of marinara sauce

## Directions:

1. Bring the water to a boil, add the quinoa and reduce heat to medium low. Let it simmer for 12-15 minutes until tender and then let it stand for 5 minutes. Fluff with fork when ready to serve.

2. Heat the two teaspoons of coconut oil in a large skillet over a medium-high heat. Add the shrimp, stirring occasionally for 7-10 minutes until cooked. Transfer to a plate and set aside.

3. Heat the remaining oil in the same pan over a medium-high heat. Add the onion and garlic, and cook for two minutes before adding the broccoli. Cover the pan with a lid and let it cook for 5-10 minutes, checking the broccoli until it is tender.

4. Add the sauce and shrimp, and cook until the sauce thickens slightly.

5. Serve warm with the quinoa on the side.

*NUTRITION FACTS (PER SERVING)*

Total Carbohydrates: 50g
Dietary Fiber: 10g
Protein: 27g
Total Fat: 11g
Calories: 397

# Mexican Salad Bowl

**Preparation time:** 15 minutes
**Cooking time:** 0 minutes
**Makes:** 2 servings

## Ingredients:

1 large handful of baby salad greens
½ cup of canned black beans
½ cup of carrots, shredded
¼ cup of sweetcorn kernels
¼ cup of green onion, chopped
¼ of an avocado, diced
½ cup of salsa
2 organic pasture-raised eggs, hardboiled and chopped

## Directions:

1. In a large bowl, toss all of the ingredients together except the salsa.

2. Serve with the salsa on the side.

## Nutrition Facts (per serving)

Total Carbohydrates: 27g
Dietary Fiber: 8g
Protein: 11g
Total Fat: 9g
Calories: 219

# Healthy Vegetarian Tacos

**Preparation time:** 5 minutes
**Cooking time:** 10 minutes
**Makes:** 4 servings (2 tacos per serving)

## Ingredients:

1 (15.5 ounce) can of black beans
1 tomato, chopped
1 (1.13 ounce) organic taco seasoning
8 gluten free taco shell
1 cup of spinach
1 avocado, sliced
1 tablespoon of olive oil

## Directions:

1. Start by sautéing your spinach with half the olive oil just until the spinach begins to wilt. Set aside.

2. Add the remaining olive oil to another pan over a low heat, and add the black beans, chopped tomato, and taco seasoning. Cook for 5 minutes.

3. Add in the spinach.

4. Spoon the mixture into shells, and top with the sliced avocado.

## Nutrition Facts (per serving)

Total Carbohydrates: 50g
Dietary Fiber: 14g
Protein: 12g
Total Fat: 14g
Calories: 363

# Cauliflower Pizza

**Preparation time:** 20 minutes
**Cooking time:** 20 minutes
**Makes:** 3 servings

## Ingredients:

1 head of cauliflower
1 organic pasture-raised egg
1 teaspoon of Italian seasoning
1/8 teaspoon of salt

1 teaspoon of garlic powder
½ cup of dairy-free organic pesto
½ cup of marinara sauce
1 handful of fresh basil

## Directions:

1. Preheat oven to 400°F.

2. Starting by steaming the cauliflower in a quarter of a cup of water for 5 minutes. Transfer the cauliflower to a food processor, and blend until it is finely chopped, almost like rice.

3. Place the cauliflower into a nut milk bag or cheese cloth, and wring out all of the water.

4. Put the cauliflower into a mixing bowl and add in the egg, seasoning, salt, pepper and garlic powder. Mix until combined.

5. Transfer to a pizza pan or a baking sheet, flatten out and bake for 15 minutes.

6. Take the pizza crust out, and top with the sauce and pesto. Bake for another 20 minutes.

7. Top with fresh basil.

## Nutrition Facts (per serving)

Total Carbohydrates: 17g
Dietary Fiber: 5g
Protein: 10g
Total Fat: 23g
Calories: 296

# Tuna Veggie Wrap

**Preparation time:** 10 minutes
**Cooking time:** 0 minutes
**Makes:** 1 serving

## Ingredients:

1 (6 ounce) can of wild tuna
1 gluten-free tortilla
¼ cup of grape tomatoes, halved
¼ of a cucumber, sliced
3 sprigs of fresh cilantro, chopped
1 tablespoon of avocado-based mayonnaise (use an olive oil based if you cannot find avocado-based)
1 teaspoon of sriracha sauce

## Directions:

1. Place the tortilla on a large serving plate, and spread on the avocado mayonnaise, sriracha sauce and the tuna.

2. Add the tomatoes, cucumber and cilantro.

3. Roll into a wrap, and enjoy.

## Nutrition Facts (per serving)

Total Carbohydrates: 28g
Dietary Fiber: 2g
Protein: 47g
Total Fat: 16g
Calories: 459

# Turmeric Brown Rice With Shrimp

**Preparation time:** 5 minutes
**Cooking time:** 35 minutes
**Makes:** 4 servings

## Ingredients:

2 cups of uncooked brown rice
4 cups of organic low-sodium vegetable broth
1 teaspoon of ground turmeric
1 pound of peeled shrimp
Salt to taste
1 tablespoon of olive oil for cooking

## Directions:

1. Bring the rice and the vegetable broth to a boil, and cook for about 35 minutes.

2. While the rice is cooking, heat a medium skillet over a medium heat, and add the olive oil. Cook the shrimp until they are well done.

3. Add the turmeric and salt to the pot of cooked rice, and stir until combined.

4. Divide the rice between four plates and top with the cooked shrimp.

## Nutrition Facts (per serving)

Total Carbohydrates: 74g
Dietary Fiber: 6g
Protein: 25g
Total Fat: 7g
Calories: 470

# Protein-Packed Zoodles

**Preparation time:** 5 minutes
**Cooking time:** 15 minutes
**Makes:** 6 servings

## Ingredients:

1 and a ½ cups of organic low-sodium vegetable broth
½ cup of dry lentils, rinsed
1 cup of basil leaves
1 garlic clove
¼ cup of walnuts
¼ cup of olive oil
¼ cup of water
4 zucchinis
8 large mushrooms, sliced

## Directions:

1. Cook the lentils in the vegetable broth for about 15 minutes.

2. Place the basil, walnuts, garlic and olive oil into a food processor, and blend. Slowly add in water to thin out the pesto to the desired consistency.

3. Using a spiralizer, turn the zucchinis into noodles, and top with the pesto.

4. Cook the mushrooms in a pan over a medium heat until they are softened. Add the mushrooms to the zucchini noodles, and top with the cooked lentils.

## Nutrition Facts (per serving)

Total Carbohydrates: 16g
Dietary Fiber: 6g
Protein: 7g
Total Fat: 12g
Calories: 187

# Beans & Greens Salad

**Preparation time:** 10 minutes
**Cooking time:** 45 minutes
**Makes:** 6 servings

## Ingredients:

1 cup of dry lima beans
1 cup of pitted olives
½ of a yellow onion, sliced
6 tablespoons of olive oil
2 cups of kale
4 anchovies

## Directions:

1. Bring 3 cups of water and lima beans to a boil, and cook for 40 minutes. Once cooked, drain and rinse the beans and set aside.

2. In a food processor or blender, blend the olives and onions until finely chopped.

3. In a large skillet, heat 2 tablespoons of the olive oil over medium heat, add the onion mixture, and then add the kale and anchovies. Sauté for about 3 minutes. Stir in the beans.

4. Serve warm, with the additional 4 tablespoons of olive oil.

## Nutrition Facts (per serving)

Total Carbohydrates: 24g
Dietary Fiber: 8g
Protein: 10g
Total Fat: 51g
Calories: 582

# Salmon Skewers

**Preparation time:** 10 minutes
**Cooking time:** 25 minutes
**Makes:** 8 servings

## Ingredients:

½ cup of olive oil
1 garlic clove, minced
1 tablespoon of fresh mint, chopped
¾ pound of salmon, skin and bones removed, cubed
12 cremini mushrooms, halved
1 head of broccoli florets
Sea salt to taste
8 wooden skewers

## Directions:

1. Preheat oven to 375°F.

2. In a bowl, combine the olive oil, garlic, mint and salt.

3. Combine the salmon, mushrooms and broccoli in a baking dish, drizzle with the marinade, and toss until the salmon is well covered.

4. Layer the salmon, mushrooms and broccoli on the skewers in any order.

5. Cook the skewers on a broiling pan for 25 minutes, being sure to turn them halfway through.

## Nutrition Facts (per serving)

Total Carbohydrates: 6g
Dietary Fiber: 2g
Protein: 12g
Total Fat: 16g
Calories: 21

# Teriyaki Lettuce Wraps

**Preparation time:** 10 minutes
**Cooking time:** 7 minutes
**Makes:** 3 servings

## Ingredients:

- 1 cup of cooked brown rice
- 2 Tbsp. coconut aminos)
- 1 tablespoon of rice vinegar
- 1 teaspoon of ground ginger
- 1 carrot, thinly sliced
- 1 tablespoon of olive oil
- 1 head of lettuce

## Directions:

1. Place the coconut aminos, rice vinegar, and ground ginger in a small bowl, and whisk. Add the brown rice and stir.

2. Scoop the mixture into three large lettuce leaves, and serve as you would a taco.

## Nutrition Facts (per serving)

Total Carbohydrates: 23g
Dietary Fiber: 4g
Protein: 4g
Total Fat: 5g
Calories: 154

# Rice Bowls

**Preparation time:** 10 minutes
**Cooking time:** 0 minutes
**Makes:** 2 servings

## Ingredients:

1 cup of cooked brown rice
½ cup of canned black beans, drained
1 tomato, chopped
1 handful of fresh parsley
1 tablespoon of tahini
Sea salt to taste

## Directions:

1. Place the cooked brown rice in a large serving bowl, and top with the rest of the ingredients. Drizzle with tahini, and a pinch of sea salt.

2. Divide between two bowls.

## Nutrition Facts (per serving)

Total Carbohydrates: 37g
Dietary Fiber: 7g
Protein: 8g
Total Fat: 5g
Calories: 219

# Coconut Quinoa Stir Fry

**Preparation time:** 10 minutes
**Cooking time:** 25 minutes
**Makes:** 2 servings

## Ingredients:

1 cup of uncooked quinoa, rinsed
1 and a ½ cups of water
½ cup of coconut milk
1 cup of broccoli, steamed
1 cup of cauliflower, steamed
2 tablespoons of coconut oil, melted
Sea salt to taste

## Directions:

1. Place the rinsed quinoa into a large pot with the water and coconut milk. Bring to a boil, and then simmer for 20-25 minutes.

2. While the quinoa is cooking, steam the broccoli and cauliflower in a small amount of water until tender.

3. Serve the quinoa with half a cup of broccoli and half a cup of cauliflower per serving, drizzle with coconut oil, and add a pinch of salt.

## Nutrition Facts (per serving)

Total Carbohydrates: 63g
Dietary Fiber: 11g
Protein: 15g
Total Fat: 33g
Calories: 589

# Quinoa Tacos

**Preparation time:** 15 minutes
**Cooking time:** 25 minutes
**Makes:** 4 servings (2 tacos per serving)

## Ingredients:

1 cup of uncooked quinoa, rinsed
1 packet of organic taco seasoning
1 cup of canned black beans
1 cup of pinto beans
8 large lettuce leaves

## Directions:

1. Place the rinsed quinoa into a large pot with 2 cups of water and bring to a boil, then simmer for 20-25 minutes.

2. While the quinoa is cooking, add the beans and taco seasoning to a large mixing bowl and stir to combine.

3. Add the cooked quinoa to the mixing bowl with the beans and stir.

4. Evenly divide the mixture among the lettuce leaves and enjoy.

## Nutrition Facts (per serving)

Total Carbohydrates: 47g
Dietary Fiber: 10g
Protein: 11g
Total Fat: 3g
Calories: 258

# Beet Veggie Burgers

**Preparation time:** 15 minutes
**Cooking time:** 30 minutes
**Makes:** 4 servings

## Ingredients:

2 cups of cooked brown rice
1 cup of beets, diced
¼ cup of dill, chopped
1 (15 ounce) can of black beans
1 organic pasture-raised egg
2 tablespoon of olive oil
Lettuce leaves for the "bun"

## Directions:

1. Start by preheating the oven to 375°F, and line a large baking sheet with parchment paper.

2. Combine the cooked rice with the beets, olive oil and dill.

3. Mash the black beans with the egg in a separate bowl, and then add to the rice mixture.

4. Form into 4 patties, and grill for about 8 minutes each side.

5. Create a "bun" around each patty with the lettuce leaves and serve immediately.

## Nutrition Facts (per serving)

Total Carbohydrates: 44g
Dietary Fiber: 10g
Protein: 11g
Total Fat: 9g
Calories: 297

# Butternut Squash Soup

**Preparation time:** 15 minutes
**Cooking time:** 20 minutes
**Makes:** 6 servings

## Ingredients:

2 cups of frozen organic butternut squash
1 cup of organic low-sodium vegetable broth
1 cup of coconut milk
2 tablespoons of coconut oil
½ teaspoon of cinnamon
2 garlic cloves, minced

## Directions:

1. Place all of the ingredients into a large stock pot, and bring to a boil. Simmer for 20-25 minutes.

2. Let the soup cool, and then with an immersion blender, blend until smooth.

3. Serve with a large salad for a full meal.

## Nutrition Facts (per serving)

Total Carbohydrates: 8g
Dietary Fiber: 2g
Protein: 2g
Total Fat: 14g
Calories: 155

# Chicken Marinara Squash

**Preparation time:** 10 minutes
**Cooking time:** 35 minutes
**Makes:** 2 servings

## Ingredients:

2 organic free range chicken breasts
½ cup of no added sugar low sodium marinara sauce
¼ cup of basil, chopped
3 garlic cloves, chopped
3 tablespoons of olive oil
1 medium spaghetti squash
¼ teaspoon of salt
¼ teaspoon of pepper

## Directions:

1. Start by preheating the oven to 375°F.

2. Cut the spaghetti squash in half, and drizzle with 1 tablespoon of the olive oil, the sea salt and the black pepper. Place cut side down on a sheet of parchment paper on a large baking sheet.

3. Bake the squash for 30-35 minutes, until you are able to use a fork to scrape the squash out.

4. While the squash is cooking, marinate your chicken breast with the remaining 2 tablespoons of olive oil and chopped garlic cloves. Cook your chicken breast to your liking - sauté, grill, or bake.

5. Scoop out the squash with a fork and top with the cooked chicken breast, a quarter of a cup of marinara sauce per serving and the chopped basil.

## Nutrition Facts (per serving)

Total Carbohydrates: 19g
Dietary Fiber: 4g
Protein: 29g
Total Fat: 26g
Calories: 423

# Healthy Chef Salad

**Preparation time:** 1 minute
**Cooking time:** 0 minutes
**Makes:** 1 serving

## Ingredients:

2 cups of baby greens
½ cup of canned black beans
1 tomato, diced
¼ of an avocado, diced
¼ of a red onion, chopped
1 organic pasture-raised hardboiled egg, crumbled
Juice of 1 lemon
1 teaspoon olive oil

## Directions:

1. Whisk the lemon and olive oil together to create the salad dressing.

2. Toss all of the salad ingredients together with the dressing.

## Nutrition Facts (per serving)

Total Carbohydrates: 26g
Dietary Fiber: 12g
Protein: 15g
Total Fat: 11g
Calories: 251

# Avocado Chicken Salad

**Preparation time:** 10 minutes
**Cooking time:** 15 minutes
**Makes:** 4 servings

## Ingredients:

2 cups organic free range chicken, cooked
2 medium avocados
2 tablespoons of fresh squeezed lime juice

¼ cup of green onion
½ cup of fresh cilantro
2 tablespoons of Greek yogurt

## Directions:

1. Shred the chicken until you have 2 cups of chicken shredded into fairly large chunks.

2. Dice the avocados into medium sized pieces, mix with 1 tablespoon of the lime juice, and season the avocados with salt to taste. Thinly slice the green onion and finely chop the cilantro.

3. Mix the Greek yogurt and the remaining 1 tablespoon of lime juice to make the dressing.

4. Put the chicken into a bowl large enough to hold all the salad ingredients. Add the sliced green onions and dressing and toss until all the chicken is coated with the dressing.

5. Add the avocados and any lime juice in the bottom of the bowl and gently combine with the chicken. Then, add the chopped cilantro and gently mix into the salad, just until it is barely combined.

6. Serve right away or chill for a while before serving.

## Nutrition Facts (per serving)

Total Carbohydrates: 6g
Dietary Fiber: 5g
Protein: 15g
Total Fat: 12g
Calories: 184

# Salmon Burgers

**Preparation time:** 15 minutes
**Cooking time:** 8 minutes
**Makes:** 6 servings

## Ingredients:

¾ cup of green onions, chopped
1 handful of cilantro
1 teaspoon of lemon juice
1 ½ cups of fresh spinach, chopped
1 pound of fresh water salmon
1 cup of cooked quinoa
1 teaspoon of Celtic or Himalayan sea salt
1 tablespoon of coconut oil for cooking
Lettuce leaves for the "bun"

## Directions:

1. Place all ingredients, except the coconut oil and lettuce leaves, into a food processor, and pulse until combined.

2. Form into patties, and cook on a heated skillet with coconut oil for 4 to 5 minutes each side or until cooked through

3. Serve using lettuce as your "bun".

## Nutrition Facts (per serving)

Total Carbohydrates: 0g
Dietary Fiber: 0g
Protein: 14g
Total Fat: 10g
Calories: 154

# Lentil Stew

**Preparation time:** 10 minutes
**Cooking time:** 20 minutes
**Makes:** 4 servings

## Ingredients:

1 tablespoon of coconut oil
2 sweet potatoes, diced
1 yellow onion, diced
4 cloves of garlic, minced
1 teaspoon of ground cumin
1 tablespoon of lime juice
6 cups of organic low sodium vegetable or chicken broth
1 cup of French green lentils, soaked
1 bay leaf
3 large kale leaves, stems removed, chopped

## Directions:

1. Heat a large stockpot over a medium heat, add coconut oil, sweet potato and onion. Sauté for 15 minutes, stirring occasionally.

2. Add garlic and cumin, and stir occasionally for 3 minutes.

3. Now add lime juice, vegetable stock, lentils and a bay leaf. Bring to a boil.

4. Reduce the heat to a simmer and cook, covered, for another 15 minutes. Stir in the kale and cook for a further 12 minutes. Season with salt and pepper to taste.

## Nutrition Facts (per serving)

Total Carbohydrates: 51g
Dietary Fiber: 14g
Protein: 17g
Total Fat: 4g
Calories: 30

# Salmon Nori Rolls

**Preparation time:** 10 minutes
**Cooking time:** 15 minutes
**Makes:** 1 serving

## Ingredients:

2 nori wraps
½ can of smoked wild salmon, cooked & shredded
½ cucumber, chopped
¼ of an avocado, diced
4 tablespoons of hummus
Coconut aminos for dipping

## Directions:

1.  Spread the hummus on the nori wraps, and fill with smoked wild salmon, cucumbers, and avocado.

2.  Dip in coconut aminos, and enjoy!

## Nutrition Facts (per serving)

Total Carbohydrates: 21g
Dietary Fiber: 8g
Protein: 40g
Total Fat: 23g
Calories: 447

# Asian Lettuce Wraps

**Preparation time:** 10 minutes
**Cooking time:** 15 minutes
**Makes:** 4 servings

## Ingredients:

1 head of large leaf lettuce.
1 pound of large shrimp, peeled and deveined
1 tablespoon of coconut oil
1 avocado, cubed
½ cucumber, sliced into strips
½ cup of cilantro, chopped
¼ cup of broccoli sprouts

2 tablespoons of purple cabbage, shredded
½ cup of shredded carrots
Salt and pepper to taste

### Dip:

1 teaspoon of sesame oil
¼ cup of coconut aminos
2 tablespoons of creamy peanut butter

## Directions:

1. Start by sautéing the shrimp in the coconut oil over medium heat until cooked through. Season with salt and pepper.

2. Whisk all of the ingredients for the dip together and set aside.

3. Select four large lettuce leaves to use as lettuce cups and divide the carrots, cucumber and cabbage between each lettuce cup. Top with the shrimp, cilantro, broccoli sprouts and avocado and roll up into a wrap.

4. Dip into the Asian-style peanut sauce.

## Nutrition Facts (per serving)

Total Carbohydrates: 13g
Dietary Fiber: 7g
Protein: 20g
Total Fat: 21g
Calories: 308

# Italian Style Pasta

**Preparation time:** 10 minutes
**Cooking time:** 20 minutes
**Makes:** 6 servings

## Ingredients:

1 (12 ounce) package of brown rice rigatoni pasta, cooked
½ cup of sun-dried tomatoes
½ cup of walnuts, chopped
½ cup of basil leaves
3 cloves of garlic, minced
1 teaspoon of sea salt
1 cup of roasted bell pepper strips
1 cup of mushrooms, chopped and cooked

## Directions:

1.  In a medium bowl, mix the sun-dried tomatoes with 1 cup of water and soak for 15 minutes. Remove the tomatoes but set the water aside for later.

2.  In a food processor, process the tomatoes, walnuts, basil, garlic and sea salt until smooth.

3.  Add the water used to soak the tomatoes 2 tablespoons at a time and pulse until the pesto is smooth.

4.  Scoop out the pesto and set it aside in a bowl. Stir the pesto into the pasta and mix in the bell pepper strips, and cooked mushrooms.

5.  Enjoy.

## Nutrition Facts (per serving)

Total Carbohydrates: 55g
Dietary Fiber: 5g
Protein: 12g
Total Fat: 8g
Calories: 337

# SNACK RECIPES

# Ants on a Log

**Preparation time:** 5 minutes
**Cooking time:** 0 minutes
**Makes:** 2 servings

## Ingredients:

6 celery sticks
3 tablespoons of almond butter
3 tablespoons of raisins

## Directions:

1.  Spread half a tablespoon of almond butter on each celery stick.

2.  Top with half a tablespoon of raisins on each celery stick.

3.  Divide the celery sticks between two plate, and enjoy!

## Nutrition Facts (per serving)

Total Carbohydrates: 17g
Dietary Fiber: 2g
Net Carbs:
Protein: 4g
Total Fat: 14g
Calories: 201

# Candied Dates

**Preparation time:** 5 minutes
**Cooking time:** 0 minutes
**Makes:** 2 servings

## Ingredients:

  4 pitted medjool dates
  2 tablespoons of peanut butter
  2 tablespoons of dark cocoa nibs

## Directions:

1. Slice the pitted dates in half, and spread half a tablespoon of peanut butter on each date.

2. Top each date with half a tablespoon of dark cocoa nibs.

3. Divide the candied dates between two plates, and enjoy!

## Nutrition Facts (per serving)

Total Carbohydrates: 20g
Dietary Fiber: 3g
Net Carbs:
Protein: 5g
Total Fat: 12g
Calories: 187

# Baked Sweet Potato Chips

**Preparation time:** 10 minutes
**Cooking time:** 25 minutes
**Makes:** 4 servings

## Ingredients:

2 medium sweet potatoes, peeled and thinly sliced
1 tablespoon of coconut oil, melted
½ teaspoon of sea salt

## Directions:

1. Start by preheating the oven to 400°F, and lining a large baking sheet with parchment paper.

2. Spread out the thinly sliced sweet potatoes, and drizzle with the melted coconut oil, and season with the salt.

3. Bake, flipping half way through, for 25 minutes or until the edges are crisp.

## Nutrition Facts (per serving)

Total Carbohydrates: 19g
Dietary Fiber: 3g
Net Carbs:
Protein: 2g
Total Fat: 4g
Calories: 112

# Chia Pudding

**Preparation time:** 15 minutes
**Cooking time:** 0 minutes
**Makes:** 6 servings

## Ingredients:

2 cups of full fat coconut milk
½ cup of chia seeds
1 teaspoon of pure vanilla extract
¼ cup of pure maple syrup
¼ cup of peanut butter

## Directions:

1. Place the chia seeds in a large glass mixing bowl, add the coconut milk, and whisk.

2. Add in the vanilla, pure maple syrup and peanut butter, and whisk until combined.

3. Store in the fridge overnight to allow the chia seeds to form a pudding.

## Nutrition Facts (per serving)

Total Carbohydrates: 375
Dietary Fiber: 9g
Net Carbs:
Protein: 8g
Total Fat: 31g
Calories: 375

# Berry Delight

**Preparation time:** 15 minutes
**Cooking time:** 0 minutes
**Makes:** 6 servings

## Ingredients:

1 cup of fresh organic blueberries
1 cup of fresh organic raspberries
1 cup of fresh organic blackberries
¼ cup of raw honey
1 tablespoon of cinnamon

## Directions:

1. Mix all the berries together in a large bowl, add in the honey, and gently stir.

2. Sprinkle with the cinnamon.

## Nutrition Facts (per serving)

Total Carbohydrates: 20g
Dietary Fiber: 3g
Net Carbs:
Protein: 1g
Total Fat: 0g
Calories: 78

# Pineapple Ginger Smoothie

**Preparation time:** 10 minutes
**Cooking time:** 0 minutes
**Makes:** 2 servings

## Ingredients:

2 cups of frozen pineapple
1 cup of frozen mango
1 small piece of ginger, 2 inches
1 celery stalk, chopped
2 cups of coconut water

## Directions:

1. Add all of your ingredients to a high speed blender and blend for around one minute.

2. Divide between two glasses, and enjoy immediately.

## Nutrition Facts (per serving)

Total Carbohydrates: 36g
Dietary Fiber: 4g
Net Carbs:
Protein: 1g
Total Fat: 0g
Calories: 137

# Blueberry & Chia Flax Seed Pudding

**Preparation time:** 10 minutes
**Cooking time:** 15 minutes
**Makes:** 4 servings

## Ingredients:

2 cups of almond milk
3 tablespoons of chia seeds
3 tablespoons of ground flaxseed
¼ cup of blueberries

## Directions:

1. Heat up a pan on a medium heat and add all of the ingredients except the blueberries.

2. Stir all the ingredients until the pudding is thick, this will take around 3 minutes.

3. Pour the pudding into a bowl and top with blueberries.

## Nutrition Facts (per serving)

Total Carbohydrates: 23g
Dietary Fiber: 12g
Net Carbs:
Protein: 7g
Total Fat: 15g
Calories: 243

# Spicy Roasted Chickpeas

**Preparation time:** 10 minutes
**Cooking time:** 40 minutes
**Makes:** 6 servings

## Ingredients:

2 (15 ounce) cans of chickpeas, drained and rinsed
1 teaspoon of paprika
1 teaspoon of turmeric
¼ teaspoon of cayenne pepper
2 teaspoons of coconut oil, melted

## Directions:

1. Preheat oven to 425°F.

2. Line a baking sheet with paper towels and place the chickpeas on them and use more paper towels to dry off the chickpeas as much as possible. Remove all of the paper towels.

3. Add the oil and spices to the chickpeas and mix well.

4. Roast your chickpeas for 40 minutes, stirring every 10 minutes.

5. When the chickpeas are done, remove from the oven and let completely cool.

## Nutrition Facts (per serving)

Total Carbohydrates: 19g
Dietary Fiber: 6g
Net Carbs:
Protein: 7g
Total Fat: 4g
Calories: 138

# Baked Kale Chips

**Preparation time:** 10 minutes
**Cooking time:** 10 - 20 minutes
**Makes:** 2 servings

## Ingredients:

1 bunch of kale, rinsed and dried
2 teaspoons of olive oil
Sea salt and pepper to taste

## Directions:

1.  Preheat oven to 400°F.

2.  Rinse kale and tear into small pieces.

3.  Place the kale on a large cooking sheet.

4.  Drizzle the olive oil all over the kale and season with salt and pepper.

5.  Bake in the oven for 10-20 minutes. The kale chips will be done when they are light and crisp.

## Nutrition Facts (per serving)

Total Carbohydrates: 3g
Dietary Fiber: 1g
Net Carbs:
Protein: 1g
Total Fat: 5g
Calories: 56

# Berry Energy Bites

**Preparation time:** 10 minutes
**Cooking time:** 0 minutes
**Makes:** 6 servings

## Ingredients:

½ cup of coconut flour
1 teaspoon of cinnamon
1 tablespoon of coconut sugar
¼ cup of dried blueberries
½ - 1 cup of almond milk

## Directions:

1. In a large mixing bowl, add the coconut flour, cinnamon, coconut sugar and blueberries, and mix well.

2. Add the almond milk slowly until a firm dough is formed.

3. Form into bite sized balls and refrigerate for 30 minutes so they can harden up.

4. Store leftovers in the refrigerator.

## Nutrition Facts (per serving)

Total Carbohydrates: 18g
Dietary Fiber: 1g
Net Carbs:
Protein: 1g
Total Fat: 1g
Calories: 80

# Quinoa & Spinach Egg Bites

**Preparation time:** 10 minutes
**Cooking time:** 20 minutes
**Makes:** 4 servings

## Ingredients:

1 cup of cooked quinoa
2 large organic pasture-raised eggs
1/3 cup of chopped spinach
1 tablespoon of chopped parsley
Salt and pepper to taste

## Directions:

1. Preheat oven to 350°F and grease a muffin tin with coconut oil.

2. Mix the quinoa, eggs, parsley, spinach, salt and pepper until everything is combined.

3. Spoon the mixture into the muffin tins, filling them to the top.

4. Bake for 20 minutes.

## Nutrition Facts (per serving)

Total Carbohydrates: 14g
Dietary Fiber: 2g
Net Carbs:
Protein: 6g
Total Fat: 3g
Calories: 109

# Roasted Beets

**Preparation time:** 10 minutes
**Cooking time:** 35-45 minutes
**Makes:** 4 servings

## Ingredients:

2 and a ½ pounds of beets, peeled and diced
1 tablespoon of coconut oil, melted
1 teaspoon of salt

## Directions:

1. Preheat the oven to 400°F.

2. Spread the beets onto a baking sheet and drizzle with melted coconut oil.

3. Add salt and mix well.

4. Roast the beets in the oven for 35-45 minutes, until the beets are soft.

## Nutrition Facts (per serving)

Total Carbohydrates: 7g
Dietary Fiber: 2g
Net Carbs:
Protein: 1g
Total Fat: 4g
Calories: 59

# Bruschetta

**Preparation time:** 60 minutes
**Cooking time:** 0 minutes
**Makes:** 4 servings

## Ingredients:

4 medium tomatoes, diced
1 red onion, diced
¼ cup of extra virgin olive oil
2 tablespoons of balsamic vinegar
2 cloves of garlic, minced
1 teaspoon of sea salt
¼ teaspoon of ground black pepper

## Directions:

1. Place all of the ingredients into a large bowl, and stir gently.

2. Refrigerate for 1 hour before serving on gluten-free toast (toast is not included in nutritional information)

## Nutrition Facts (per serving)

Total Carbohydrates: 8g
Dietary Fiber: 2g
Net Carbs:
Protein: 1g
Total Fat: 14g
Calories: 156

# Cashew Cheese

**Preparation time:** 2 hours
**Cooking time:** 0 minutes
**Makes:** 6 servings

## Ingredients:

1 cup of raw cashews
Juice of ½ lemon
1 tablespoon of nutritional yeast
Salt and pepper to taste
¼ cup of fresh basil

## Directions:

1. Soak the cashews in 1 cup of water for 2 hours. Drain.

2. Place the cashews, lemon juice, nutritional yeast and fresh basil into a food processor and blend until smooth. Add in 1 tablespoon of water at a time to make it creamy, but not runny.

3. Season with salt and pepper and then spread it on gluten-free bread or toast.

4. Store in an airtight jar in the refrigerator.

## Nutrition Facts (per serving)

Total Carbohydrates: 126g
Dietary Fiber: 1g
Net Carbs:
Protein: 4g
Total Fat: 10g
Calories: 126

# Acai Smoothie Bowl

**Preparation time:** 15 minutes
**Cooking time:** 0 minutes
**Makes:** 1 serving

## Ingredients:

- 2 packets frozen acai berries
- 1 cup of unsweetened almond milk
- ½ a frozen banana
- 4 frozen strawberries
- 2 tablespoons of protein powder

## Directions:

1. Place all ingredients into a high speed blender, and blend until smooth.

2. Empty the mixture into a bowl and eat with a spoon like ice-cream.

## Nutrition Facts (per serving)

Total Carbohydrates: 43g
Dietary Fiber: 8g
Net Carbs:
Protein: 4g
Total Fat: 4g
Calories: 201

# SIDES, SAUCES & DRESSINGS RECIPES

# Avocado Vinaigrette

**Preparation time:** 10 minutes
**Cooking time:** 0 minutes
**Makes:** 8 servings

## Ingredients:

1 avocado
¼ cup of white wine vinegar
Juice of two lemons
½ cup of extra virgin olive oil
Salt and pepper to taste

## Directions:

1. In a food processor or blender, combine all of the ingredients and blend until smooth and creamy.

2. Store in the fridge in an air-tight container

## Nutrition Facts (per serving)

Total Carbohydrates: 1g
Dietary Fiber: 1g
Net Carbs:
Protein: 0g
Total Fat: 16g
Calories: 148

# Lemon Garlic Brussel Sprouts

**Preparation time:** 10 minutes
**Cooking time:** 25 minutes
**Makes:** 6 servings

## Ingredients:

  2 pounds of Brussels sprouts, halved
  3 tablespoons of avocado oil
  5 cloves of garlic, chopped
  1 large lemon, zest and juice
  Salt and pepper to taste

## Directions:

1.  In a large skillet, heat the avocado oil over a medium-high heat.

2.  Add Brussels sprouts and sauté for around 20 minutes until they are tender.

3.  Add the garlic and the lemon zest and juice.

4.  Season with salt and pepper to taste.

## Nutrition Facts (per serving)

Total Carbohydrates: 3
Dietary Fiber: 1g
Net Carbs:
Protein: 1
Total Fat: 7g
Calories: 72

# Turmeric Bites

**Preparation time:** 10 minutes
**Cooking time:** 0 minutes
**Makes:** 6 servings

## Ingredients:

1/3 cup of ground turmeric
3 tablespoons of raw honey
1 tablespoon of coconut oil

## Directions:

1. Line a plate or baking sheet with parchment paper.

2. Heat up the honey and coconut oil a little bit if the coconut oil is solid.

3. Stir together all of your ingredients and then make small balls out of the mixture.

4. Place your balls on the baking sheet and freeze for around 10 minutes.

5. Once the turmeric bites are frozen, store them in the fridge or freezer.

## Nutrition Facts (per serving)

Total Carbohydrates: 12g
Dietary Fiber: 1g
Net Carbs:
Protein: 0g
Total Fat: 3g
Calories: 72

# Broccoli Quinoa Salad

**Preparation time:** 10 minutes
**Cooking time:** 20 minutes
**Makes:** 4 servings

## Ingredients:

2 cups of cooked quinoa
1 cup of grape tomatoes, halved
½ head of broccoli, chopped
2 tablespoons of walnuts
1 lemon, juiced

## Directions:

1. In a medium bowl, toss all of the ingredients.

2. Season with salt and pepper to taste.

## Nutrition Facts (per serving)

Total Carbohydrates: 35g
Dietary Fiber: 6g
Protein: 9g
Total Fat: 5g
Calories: 208

# Broccoli & Potato Soup

**Preparation time:** 10 minutes
**Cooking time:** 30 minutes
**Makes:** 4 servings

## Ingredients:

1 tablespoon of olive oil
1 small onion, diced
2 cloves of garlic, minced
1 head of broccoli
2 large potatoes, peeled and quartered
3 cups of organic low sodium vegetable broth
Salt and pepper to taste

## Directions:

1. In a large pot, heat the olive oil and cook the onions and garlic over a medium heat until the onions are translucent.

2. Add the vegetable broth, potatoes and broccoli to the pot. Cover and bring to a boil. Cook for around 15 minutes, until the potatoes are tender.

3. Puree the soup in a blender.

4. Season with salt and pepper to taste.

## Nutrition Facts (per serving)

Total Carbohydrates: 32g
Dietary Fiber: 7g
Net Carbs:
Protein: 8g
Total Fat: 4g
Calories: 183

# Anti-Inflammatory Dressing

**Preparation time:** 10 minutes
**Cooking time:** 0 minutes
**Makes:** 4 servings

## Ingredients:

¼ cup of raw cashews
2/3 cup of cashew milk
1 tablespoon of apple cider vinegar
1 tablespoon of agave nectar
½ teaspoon of ground turmeric
½ teaspoon of fresh minced ginger
¼ teaspoon of Dijon mustard
Salt and pepper to taste

## Directions:

1. Place the cashews in a food processor or high speed blender and grind into a powder.

2. Add the remaining ingredients and puree for about a minute, or until nice and smooth. Taste, and adjust seasonings as needed.

3. Chill for 30 minutes and then stir the dressing before pouring on the salad.

## Nutrition Facts (per serving)

Total Carbohydrates: 8g
Dietary Fiber: 0g
Net Carbs:
Protein: 2g
Total Fat: 4g
Calories: 74

# Turmeric Cauliflower

**Preparation time:** 10 minutes
**Cooking time:** 25 - 30 minutes
**Makes:** 3 servings

## Ingredients:

1 large cauliflower head
2 teaspoons of turmeric
3 tablespoons olive oil
Salt to taste

## Directions:

1. Preheat oven to 400°F.

2. Coat the cauliflower florets with the turmeric, salt and olive oil.

3. Place all of the ingredients on a cookie sheet and spread so they are not on top of each other.

4. Bake for 25 - 30 minutes.

## Nutrition Facts (per serving)

Total Carbohydrates: 10g
Dietary Fiber: 4g
Net Carbs:
Protein: 4g
Total Fat: 14g
Calories: 168

# Honey Roasted Carrots

**Preparation time:** 5 minutes
**Cooking time:** 30 minutes
**Makes:** 3 servings

## Ingredients:

1 large bunch of carrots, scrubbed
2 tablespoons of olive oil
1 tablespoon of raw honey
½ teaspoon of sea salt

## Directions:

1. Preheat oven to 400°F, and line a large baking sheet with parchment paper.

2. Combine the carrots, olive oil, honey and salt in a large mixing bowl, and toss.

3. Arrange on the baking sheet and cook for 30 minutes.

## Nutrition Facts (per serving)

Total Carbohydrates: 19g
Dietary Fiber: 4g
Net Carbs:
Protein: 1g
Total Fat: 9g
Calories: 156

# Lemon Vinaigrette

**Preparation time: 5 minutes**
**Cooking time: 0 minutes**
**Makes: 3 servings**

## Ingredients:

2 tablespoons of balsamic vinegar
2 tablespoons of fresh lemon juice
½ teaspoon of sea salt
1 tablespoon of raw honey
¼ cup of olive oil

## Directions:

1. Place all of the ingredients into a bowl, and whisk.

2. Drizzle over your favorite anti-inflammatory salad.

## Nutrition Facts (per serving)

Total Carbohydrates: 8g
Dietary Fiber: 0g
Net Carbs:
Protein: 0g
Total Fat: 18g
Calories: 190

# Gingery Spice Salad Dressing

**Preparation time:** 5 minutes
**Cooking time:** 0 minutes
**Makes:** 3 servings

## Ingredients:

- ½ teaspoon of ground fresh ginger
- 1 tablespoon of raw honey
- ½ teaspoon of curry powder
- ½ teaspoon of ground turmeric
- 1 tablespoon of apple cider vinegar
- ¾ cup of full fat coconut milk

## Directions:

1. Simply place all ingredients into a blender, and blend until smooth.

2. Drizzle over your favorite anti-inflammatory salad.

## Nutrition Facts (per serving)

Total Carbohydrates: 9g
Dietary Fiber: 1g
Net Carbs:
Protein: 1g
Total Fat: 14g
Calories: 161

# Turmeric Salad Dressing

**Preparation time:** 5 minutes
**Cooking time:** 0 minutes
**Makes:** 3 servings

## Ingredients:

4 tablespoons of olive oil
Juice of 2 lemons
1 clove of garlic
1 tablespoon of ground turmeric
1 tablespoon of raw honey
Pinch of sea salt to taste

## Directions:

1. Simply place all ingredients into a blender, and blend until smooth.

2. Drizzle over your favorite anti-inflammatory salad.

## Nutrition Facts (per serving)

Total Carbohydrates: 8g
Dietary Fiber: 1g
Net Carbs:
Protein: 0g
Total Fat: 18g
Calories: 190

# Garlicy Walnut Dip

**Preparation time:** 10 minutes
**Cooking time:** 0 minutes
**Makes:** 8 servings

## Ingredients:

½ cup of walnuts
½ cup of gluten-free bread crumbs
4 cloves of garlic
1 tablespoon of lemon juice
1 tablespoon of olive oil
¾ cup of water

## Directions:

1. Add all of the ingredients to a blender, and blend until smooth.

2. Serve with fresh vegetables or gluten-free pita chips

## Nutrition Facts (per serving)

Total Carbohydrates: 6g
Dietary Fiber: 1g
Net Carbs:
Protein: 2g
Total Fat: 7g
Calories: 93

# Bean Tuna Salad

**Preparation time:** 10 minutes
**Cooking time:** 0 minutes
**Makes:** 3 servings

## Ingredients:

1 can (15.5 ounce) of cannellini beans, drained and rinsed
1 (5-6 ounce) can of tuna
1 cup of curly parsley, chopped
¼ cup of onion, finely diced
3 tablespoons of olive oil

## Directions:

1. Place the beans and tuna into a large mixing bowl, and mix well.

2. Stir in the parsley, onion, and olive oil.

3. Serve as a side dish for an extra dose of protein!

## Nutrition Facts (per serving)

Total Carbohydrates: 32g
Dietary Fiber: 7g
Net Carbs:
Protein: 25g
Total Fat: 15g
Calories: 356

# Vegetable Soup

**Preparation time:** 10 minutes
**Cooking time:** 25 minutes
**Makes:** 4 servings

## Ingredients:

1 onion, peeled and minced
1 teaspoon of turmeric
1 teaspoon of ginger
1 teaspoon of mustard powder
1 teaspoon of curry powder
½ teaspoon of cinnamon
½ teaspoon of cayenne
1 and a ½ cups of organic low sodium vegetable broth
3 cloves of garlic, minced
1 can of white beans

## Directions:

1. Simply place all the ingredients, except for the beans, into a large stock pot, and simmer for 20 minutes.

2. Add in the beans, and let the soup simmer for an additional 5 minutes.

3. Serve warm.

## Nutrition Facts (per serving)

Total Carbohydrates: 26g
Dietary Fiber: 6g
Net Carbs:
Protein: 9g
Total Fat: 1g
Calories: 142

# Butternut Squash Soup

**Preparation time:** 10 minutes
**Cooking time:** 30 minutes
**Makes:** 3 servings

## Ingredients:

1 cup of butternut squash, cubed
1 large onion
4 garlic cloves
½ cup of canned coconut milk
1 teaspoon of turmeric
1 cup of organic low sodium vegetable broth

## Directions:

1. Place all of the ingredients into a large stock pot, and simmer for 25-30 minutes, or until the squash is tender.

2. Serve warm.

## Nutrition Facts (per serving)

Total Carbohydrates: 11g
Dietary Fiber: 2g
Net Carbs:
Protein: 3g
Total Fat: 10g
Calories: 132

# DESSERT RECIPES

# Brain-Boosting Cocoa Bites

**Preparation time:** 10 minutes
**Cooking time:** 0 minutes
**Makes:** 12 servings

## Ingredients:

8 dates, pitted and coarsely chopped
2/3 cup of raw cocoa powder
1 cup of shredded coconut
2 tablespoons of water
2 cups of walnuts
1 tablespoon of coconut oil

## Directions:

1. Add all of the ingredients to a food processor or high speed blender, and blend until the mixture is well combined. Add 1 teaspoon of water at a time to bring the mixture together.

2. Remove the mixture from the blender, and roll into 1 inch balls.

3. Refrigerate until firm, and enjoy!

## Nutrition Facts (per serving)

Total Carbohydrates: 8g
Dietary Fiber: 3g
Net Carbs:
Protein: 4g
Total Fat: 33g
Calories: 318

# Anti-Inflammatory Brownies

**Preparation time:** 10 minutes
**Cooking time:** 30 minutes
**Makes:** 8 servings

## Ingredients:

1 cup of sweet potato puree
½ cup of canned black beans
2 organic pasture-raised eggs
½ cup of pure maple syrup
½ teaspoon of sea salt
½ cup of rice flour
½ cup of cocoa powder
½ cup of unsweetened almond milk
½ cup of dark chocolate cocoa nibs
½ cup of coconut oil
Coconut oil for baking

## Directions:

1. Preheat oven to 375°F, and oil a 9 inch baking dish with coconut oil.

2. In a large mixing bowl, combine all of the wet ingredients together, and then add in the dry ingredients. Whisk together until well combined.

3. Pour the mixture into the baking dish, and cook for 30 minutes.

## Nutrition Facts (per serving)

Total Carbohydrates: 23g
Dietary Fiber: 4g
Net Carbs:
Protein: 4g
Total Fat: 19g
Calories: 258

# Blueberry Energy Bites

**Preparation time:** 10 minutes
**Cooking time:** 0 minutes
**Makes:** 6 servings

## Ingredients:

½ cup of gluten-free oat flour
¼ teaspoon of cinnamon
2 tablespoons of pure maple syrup
2 tablespoons of organic peanut butter
½ teaspoon of sea salt
2 tablespoons of dried blueberries
½ cup of unsweetened almond milk

## Directions:

1. Place the dry ingredients into a mixing bowl, including the peanut butter, and stir until combined.

2. Add in the almond milk and maple syrup, and stir.

3. Form into 1 inch balls, and place in the refrigerator to firm up before serving.

## Nutrition Facts (per serving)

Total Carbohydrates: 13g
Dietary Fiber: 1g
Net Carbs:
Protein: 3g
Total Fat: 1g
Calories: 93

# Inflammation-Busting Hot Cocoa

**Preparation time:** 5 minutes
**Cooking time:** 5 minutes
**Makes:** 1 serving

## Ingredients:

½ cup of canned coconut milk
¼ teaspoon of cinnamon
1 tablespoon of pure maple syrup
1 tablespoon of raw cocoa powder
¼ teaspoon of turmeric

## Directions:

1. Place all of the ingredients into a medium pot over low heat, and whisk. Whisk over low heat for 5 minutes, being careful not to bring to a boil.

2. Serve warm.

## Nutrition Facts (per serving)

Total Carbohydrates: 37g
Dietary Fiber: 4g
Net Carbs:
Protein: 4g
Total Fat: 29g
Calories: 393

# Decadent Guilt-Free Cocoa Pudding

**Preparation time:** 10 minutes
**Cooking time:** 0 minutes
**Makes:** 1 serving

## Ingredients:

½ a ripe avocado
1 medium, super ripe banana
¼ cup of pitted medjool dates
1 tablespoon of raw cocoa powder
2 tablespoons of raw honey
¼ cup of filtered water

## Directions:

1. Place all of the ingredients into a high speed blender, and blend until super smooth. Add a teaspoon of water at a time if the consistency needs to be thinned out.

2. Serve in glass cups, or small dessert bowls, and top with walnuts, strawberries or raw cocoa nibs.

## Nutrition Facts (per serving)

Total Carbohydrates: 98g
Dietary Fiber: 12g
Net Carbs:
Protein: 5g
Total Fat: 11g
Calories: 457

# Coconut Butter Fudge

**Preparation time:** 10 minutes
**Cooking time:** 0 minutes
**Makes:** 6 servings

## Ingredients:

- 1 cup of coconut butter
- 2 tablespoons of raw honey
- ¼ teaspoon of salt
- 1 teaspoon of pure vanilla extract

## Directions:

1. Start by lining an 8 x 8 inch baking dish with parchment paper.

2. Melt the coconut butter, honey and vanilla over a low heat.

3. Pour the mixture into the baking pan, and refrigerate for 2 hours before serving.

## Nutrition Facts (per serving)

Total Carbohydrates: 6g
Dietary Fiber: 0g
Net Carbs:
Protein: 0g
Total Fat: 36g
Calories: 334

# Chocolate Fudge Bites

**Preparation time:** 10 minutes
**Cooking time:** 3 minutes
**Makes:** 10 servings

## Ingredients:

1 and a ¼ cup of boiling water
3 tablespoons of grass-fed gelatin
½ cup of cold water
½ cup of raw cocoa powder
½ cup of coconut milk powder
1 cup of coconut oil
1/3 cup of pure maple syrup

## Directions:

1. Mix one and a quarter cup of boiling water with the gelatin, and boil for 3 minutes. Then, place the gelatin mixture into a blender with the cold water and remaining ingredients. Blend for a couple of minutes to help the gelatin solidify.

2. Pour the mixture into the bottom of a greased baking dish, and refrigerate until firm.

3. Cut into small serving squares.

## Nutrition Facts (per serving)

Total Carbohydrates: 30g
Dietary Fiber: 3g
Net Carbs:
Protein: 2g
Total Fat: 24g
Calories: 317

# Raspberry Gummies

**Preparation time:** 5 minutes
**Cooking time:** 15 minutes
**Makes:** 12 servings (2 gummies each)

## Ingredients:

1 cup of frozen raspberries
3 tablespoons of raw honey
¼ cup of grass-fed gelatin
¾ cup of cold water

## Directions:

1. Place the water and frozen raspberries into a blender, and blend until smooth. Pour into a large saucepan over a medium heat.
2. Add the honey and gelatin and whisk together. Turn the heat down to low, and whisk for another 5 minutes.
3. Pour into molds or a baking dish, and place in the refrigerator for at least 1 hour until firm. If you use a baking dish, cut the gelatin into squares; if not, just pop the gelatin out of the molds.

## Nutrition Facts (per serving)

Total Carbohydrates: 9g
Dietary Fiber: 1g
Net Carbs:
Protein: 0g
Total Fat: 0g
Calories: 37

# Turmeric Milkshake

**Preparation time:** 5 minutes
**Cooking time:** 0 minutes
**Makes:** 2 servings

## Ingredients:

2 cups of unsweetened almond milk
3 tablespoons of raw honey
2 tablespoons of raw cocoa powder
1 tablespoon of ground flaxseeds
1 teaspoon of turmeric
2 frozen bananas

## Directions:

1. Place all ingredients into a high speed blender, and blend until smooth.
2. Divide between two serving glasses, and enjoy straight away.

## Nutrition Facts (per serving)

Total Carbohydrates: 74g
Dietary Fiber: 7g
Protein: 4g
Total Fat: 6g
Calories: 334

# No Bake Carrot Cake Bites

**Preparation time:** 15 minutes
**Cooking time:** 0 minutes
**Makes:** 6 servings

## Ingredients:

- 1 and a ½ cups of carrots
- 1 cup of pitted medjool dates
- ½ teaspoon of ground ginger
- 1 tablespoon of pure maple syrup
- 1 teaspoon of cinnamon
- 1 cup of walnuts
- ¾ cup of shredded coconut

## Directions:

1. Place all of the ingredients into a high speed blender or food processor, and blend until the mixture comes together, adding a teaspoon of water at a time if needed.
2. Take the carrot mixture and press down into a cupcake tin, and refrigerate until firm.
3. Pop the carrot cakes out of the muffin tin, and enjoy!

## Nutrition Facts (per serving)

Total Carbohydrates: 32g
Dietary Fiber: 5g
Net Carbs:
Protein: 3g
Total Fat: 12g
Calories: 231

# Baking Conversion Chart

## Spoon, Cups, Liquid - ml

| | |
|---|---|
| ¼ tsp. | 1.25 ml |
| 1/2 tsp. | 2.5 ml |
| 1 tsp. | 5 ml |
| 1 Tbsp. | 15 ml |
| ¼ cup | 60 ml |
| 1/3 cup | 80 ml |
| ½ cup | 125 ml |
| 1 cup | 250 ml |

## Dry Measurements

| | |
|---|---|
| 1 Tbsp. | ½ ounce |
| 1/4 cup | 2 ounces |
| 1/3 cup | 2.6 ounces |
| ½ cup | 4 ounces |
| ¾ cup | 6 ounces |
| 1 cup | 8 ounces |
| 2 cups | 16 ounces |

## Volume Liquid

| | | |
|---|---|---|
| 2 Tbsp. | 1 fl. oz. | 30 ml |
| 1/4 cup | 2 fl. oz. | 60 ml |
| ½ cup | 4 fl. oz. | 125 ml |
| 1 cup | 8 fl. oz. | 250 ml |
| 1 ½ cups | 12 fl. oz. | 375 ml |
| 2 cups/1 pint | 16 fl. oz. | 500 ml |
| 4 cups/1 quart | 32 fl. oz. | 1000 ml/ 1 liter |

# References:

1. ILSI Europe, 2015, Controlling Inflammation to Reduce Chronic Disease Risk, https://www.sciencedaily.com/releases/2015/08/150807092555.htm, Science Daily.

2. UPI, 2013, Some Foods Help Fight Inflammation, http://www.upi.com/Health_News/2013/03/24/Some-foods-help-fight-inflammation/UPI-76451364180100/

3. Nordqvist C, 2015, Medical News Today, Inflammation: Causes, Symptoms and Treatment, http://www.medicalnewstoday.com/articles/248423.php

4. WHO, 2002, Physical inactivity a leading cause of disease and disability, warns WHO, http://www.who.int/mediacentre/news/releases/release23/en/

5. Fries, W.C, 2011, WebMD, 13 Ways to Fight Sugar Cravings, http://www.webmd.com/diet/features/13-ways-to-fight-sugar-cravings#1

6. Dr. Weil, Dr. Weil's Anti-Inflammatory Food Pyramid, accessed 10 March 2017, https://www.drweil.com/diet-nutrition/anti-inflammatory-diet-pyramid/dr-weils-anti-inflammatory-food-pyramid-2-2-2/

7. Zelman, K.M, WebMD, Fiber: How Much Do You Need?, accessed 14 March 2017, http://www.webmd.com/diet/guide/fiber-how-much-do-you-need#1